Praise for Re

Amrita touches into a deep place of healing personal and collective wounding as a powerful and positive guide on the path to sexual healing and awakening. As you take her unique and inspirational journey, you will be guided to new heights of expansion and aliveness with joyful compassion.

-Rachael Jayne Groover, best-selling author of *Powerful and Feminine* and Creator of Art of Feminine Presence®

Aphrodite's Journey is a wise, generous, unflinchingly honest map home to sexual wholeness – from someone who has quite obviously walked the journey herself. Amrita Grace shares with us a unique and magical blend of clear thinking, personal details, practical exercises, expansive resources, compassion and hope. If you or someone you love is struggling in the murky aftermath of sexual abuse, this book is a welcome beacon of light and sanity.

-David Cates, respected leader in the field of sexual healing

Amrita Grace writes with authenticity, describing a journey of healing that we all must make. Sexual wholeness is a modern concept with deep, unseen and unconscious patterns. I encourage everyone to look under their own carpets in order to polish their life and their love with this easy-to-read gift from a priestess of healing".

-Caroline Muir, best-selling author of *Tantra Goddess, A Memoir of Sexual Awakening* and *Tantra, The Art of Conscious Loving*

Reclaiming Aphrodite is a simple, yet profound and authentic revealing of what it takes to heal sexually. This is a rare book, written not from a clinical perspective, but from a direct, first-hand experience of what it means to claim our wounds as points of power. Amrita's writing style is compassionate and direct, both of which assist the reader in relaxing and becoming more resourced on their healing journey.

-Saida Désilets, Ph.D., author of *Emergence of the Sensual Woman*

Reclaiming Aphrodite

The Journey to Sexual Wholeness

Amrita Grace

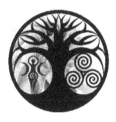

Grace Awakening Publications

Disclaimer

The information presented in this book is based on the author's personal experience of healing and recovery. It is for the purpose of education and empowerment and to assist us in individually and collectively reclaiming our birthright of sexual wholeness. The techniques explained are to be used with discretion and with the reader's liability. The author is not responsible or liable in any manner for any experiences or issues resulting from applying the techniques described in this book.

Reclaiming Aphrodite
The Journey to Sexual Wholeness

For inquiries contact: Amrita Grace
                           Grace Awakening Publications
                           PO Box 1354
                           Whittier, NC 28789
                           amrita@amritagrace.com
                           ReclaimingAphrodite.com

For every being on a path of healing

Who has the willingness and the courage

To show up for themselves

Over and over

Blessed Be!

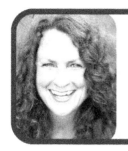

Amrita Grace

Award-Winning Author ♥ High Priestess

Certified Spiritual Sexual Educator

The Sacred Feminine Path to Wholeness®

Amrita is fiercely committed to guiding spirit-led women on a sacred, mystical, and holistic path of empowerment and wholeness. She guides them into their authentic, embodied personal power, inspiring them to live the fulfilled and abundant lives they dream of.

She's the co-founder of *The Sacred Feminine Mystery School,* leading women's retreats and certification trainings in the uniquely feminine paradigm globally celebrated as *Sacred Sexual Awakening & Healing* (AH)®

Her Certified Spiritual Sexual Educator® program trains and empowers women to professionally teach *Sacred Sexual Healing & Awakening* workshops.

Please visit her website, AmritaGrace.com, for a wide range of resources to support you on the Sacred Feminine Path to Wholeness® including the *Enchanted Chalice Blog.*

You will find resources and meditations specific to this book at AmritaGrace.com/reclaim.

Table of Contents

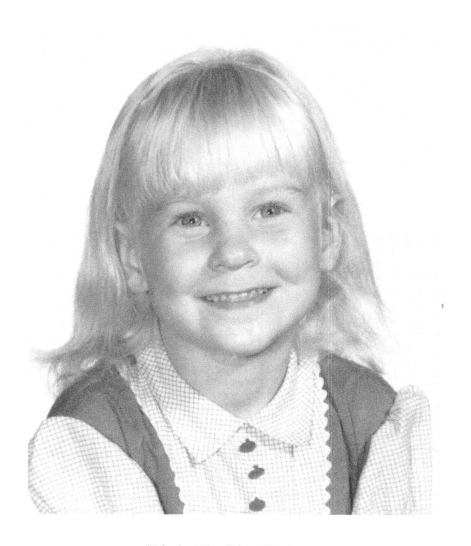

"Little Kim" in Kindergarten

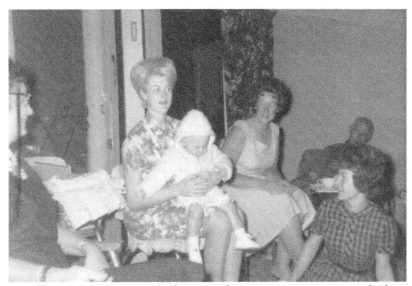

Author at age one sitting on her pregnant mom's lap,
being adored by three generations of matriarchal family:
Auntie, Grandmother, and Great Grandmother.
Grandfather is snoozing.

Chapter 1
Wholeness

Rock bottom became the solid foundation
upon which I built my life.

JK Rowling, in her 2008
commencement address to Harvard

Introduction

I am a whole, healed being. With a great deal of assistance, help, and support, I have taken a tangled knot of fragmented consciousness and lovingly unwound each thread, smoothing as I went. I have braided the threads together into a cohesive weaving with a beautiful pattern of integrated colors and textures. I love who I have become. My life is overflowing with joy. It is not without times of sadness and difficulty, for this is the human experience of contrast that we are all here to explore. Challenging times provide us with information about our inner experience so that we can make informed choices.

You are a whole, healed being. Perhaps it does not feel that way to you right now... and yet, here you are, taking a healthy step in the right direction.

We live in a very special time. A time when consciousness is on the verge of a huge leap, when more people than ever before are seeking wholeness. What does wholeness mean? Wholeness is defined as "an undivided or unbroken completeness or totality with nothing wanting." As we align ourselves with the accelerating planetary shifts, everything that is not about love is emerging to be transformed in our bodies, our energy fields, our lives, and our relationships.

You may find your own personal shadow, your pain, guilt, and fear, clamoring for integration. Your past strategies of ignoring or setting aside these parts of yourself is no longer serving you. But there are ways to liberate the neglected parts and find peace.

Embracing these lost, sad, shameful, forgotten parts of yourself is the first step in reclaiming your sexual wholeness. As you acknowledge and release that which no longer serves you, you create spaciousness for the inherent expansiveness of love to fill your being. You begin to love all of yourself, not just the shiny parts that you are projecting to the world. As you fully accept and appreciate yourself, compassion for yourself and others flows from you effortlessly.

Often, people hold shame and guilt in their sexual center, remnants of childhood events that imprinted them well before they could make informed choices. Religious doctrines, sexual abuse and trauma, and imprints of family lineages get passed down generation after generation. You can choose to shift yourself, breaking the generational patterns that unconsciously drive you. There are many tools and helping professions available to you now that were unheard of twenty years ago, and many choices for healing methods. Had I known then what I know now, my healing process would have most likely been a much shorter and easier journey.

This book specifically addresses how to successfully recover from the impact of childhood sexual abuse and is based in my own experience of healing and recovery. It is written through my own filters and perceptions of how I was impacted by my abuse and how that manifested in my adult life. Having been sexually, physically, and emotionally abused by a stepfather between the ages of five and ten, I acted out my power and self-esteem issues as an adult. Eventually, I reached the bottoming out point of deciding to turn and face my past. I self-diagnosed as a sex addict and embarked on a decade-long journey of healing and recovery. I eventually declared myself fully healed and recovered from sexual addiction. I chose methods that are considered "alternative" and rejected the mainstream approaches to recovery as unsuitable for myself. As I reflect back on the incredible beauty of the journey to wholeness that I took, it takes my breath away.

My journey eventually led me into the healing professions, first as a Reiki practitioner, then a massage therapist, and then into the realm of therapeutic somatic sexual healing. My training in these arts greatly assisted me in my own inner work, and over time I was able to achieve mastery of my sexual energy and the level of integrity that would allow me to assist others on their healing and recovery journeys. This is a perfect example of the "wounded healer" archetype. To quote the film *The Wounded Healer* by Humanity Healing Network, "Carl Jung believed that a malady of the soul could be the best possible form of training for a healer. In the search for our own cure, we discover how to help others. Wounded healers bring compassion and empathy, because they have experienced their own pain and healing process." I feel a strong resonance with these statements.

This book uses the human energy system (chakras) as a framework for the healing journey. It also includes my deeply personal accounts of some of the most painful, amazing, and magical experiences I had along the way in the form of personal short stories. I am not trained as a therapist, nor do I have a college degree. I took a very alternative path to my education as well as my recovery. What I do have to offer you is an open heart that overflows with love, compassion, and empathy for your personal process. My desire is to transmit those qualities to you as you read these pages as part of the magic of intention and energy. Please receive as much as you can, as much as you choose to, and use it for your highest and best good. This book is my love and healing offering to the world.

Igniting My Healing Journey

Personal Story: *The First Healing Steps*

Driving down the dusty dirt road on my way to Sheep Ranch, my mind wanders back to the conversation with Janine that led to this moment. "I'm hosting a women's firewalk this weekend," she said, "Would you like to come? You may find it helpful since you're just beginning your process of recovery." I replied, "Sure, why not," even though I had never been interested in such things before. Back in the present moment, I saw the turnoff to Janine's coming up, and I knew there was no turning back, either from the firewalk or from my choice to heal myself from my sexual wounding.

I arrive at the home of Janine, Jaya, and Carol around noon. They live way out in the country, with no neighbors for miles around. Large garden areas lie dormant for the winter behind deer fences. Two large buildings are visible on the property as I find a place to park my car. I head for the building that looks like a house and Janine greets me at the door. "Welcome, I'm so glad you came!" I smile shyly and go inside.

I do not know anyone here. Fifteen or so women gather in the living room, some of us sitting on the floor. I feel fearful and excited and eager. Each woman introduces herself and then Janine introduces us to Jaya, who will be taking care of the fire while we prepare to walk the coals. After some instructions about how the day will be structured, we proceed outside to the place where the fire will be built.

First, we silently build the tower of split cedar logs that

will become our coals. I remember Janine saying that the tower we build is a direct reflection of the strength of our group. We gather in a circle to honor the space where Jaya is lighting the fire. Over and over we chant, "Fire Spirit, Fire Spirit, come to the people, Fire Spirit, Fire Spirit, help us in this way!" as the paper at the bottom is slowly devoured by the licking flames. The fire begins to crackle and snap, the temperature rises, and we begin to take small steps back as the chant winds down. Once the fire is going well, Janine leads us to the temple to spend the next couple of hours preparing to walk the coals.

The other large building on the property houses the temple. As I enter the building and cross the room, I see hinged wooden shutters, which are being opened from the inside by Carol. She beckons us inside. The heady scent of sage smoke fills the air as I step down the three stairs into the temple. The carpet is light blue and very soft. A beautiful soapstone wood stove on the opposite wall gently heats the room. Along the walls of the high-ceilinged and open room are shelves filled with sculptures and images of the female form in all shapes and sizes. Animal carvings and feathers sit among the sculptures and an owl's wing hangs from the ceiling on fishing line. Drums and other instruments reside in a corner. On some level, I understand that this is a temple dedicated to the Goddess, although I have never seen such a thing before. I feel safe here, held in the arms of the ethereal feminine sacredness that permeates the room.

Janine leads the group in a series of exercises that gently help us open our hearts to each other. Over the course of several hours, these strangers begin to feel like sisters. I so want to believe that this kind of connection between people is possible. I remember the last two exercises best. "It's time for the Angel Walk," Janine announces, and smiles light the faces of those who are familiar with this process. "Line up in two rows, facing each other," she instructs, "and walk down the middle, one by one, with your eyes closed. Those of you in the rows, you may touch her very respectfully and whisper in her ears all that you appreciate about her."

I feel very nurtured and loved as I walk through the rows of women, who tell me things like, "You have such beautiful hair," and "It makes me happy just to see you smile." When the last woman completes her walk, we collapse together in a group hug as if we had been best friends since childhood. "It's time.... for the Jellyfish!" says Janine, with a twinkle in her eye and a smile on her face. "How strange," I thought, "this has all been so serious." It is serious no more as we begin to imitate her silly movements in the call and response song. We sing the chorus together, "The Jellyfish, The Jellyfish, the Jelly Fish Fish!" which leaves us all dissolved in fits of laughter.

Jaya comes in from tending the fire and instructs us on how to walk across the coals with determination and intention, eyes on the other side, keeping that goal in sight. "Walk across those coals like you MEAN IT!" she says with military precision.

The moment of truth has arrived. We file outside to a well-spread pile of coals where our tower of cedar logs has been before. Breathless fear rises in my solar plexus. We begin chanting and transmuting the fear into excitement. Women begin to walk across the 1,200 degree coals. I am one of the first few, driven by the idea that I must prove to myself, and to everyone else, that I CAN heal myself.

The coals have a soft feel to them, kind of powdery. I get to the other side feeling triumphant and ready to walk again. I walk four more times. I marvel over the fact that my feet are unmarked. We return to the temple to find some containment for our overflowing excitement and to eventually sleep. I feel that I have communed with fire and received an elemental healing. I remember one of the things that Janine said during the day: "Fire burns, except when it doesn't." I did not understand it then, but I understand it now!

I will carry the power of walking the coals with me for the rest of my life.

~

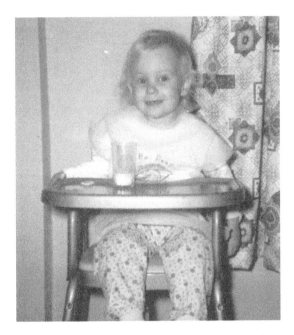

Little Kim at age two; pre-wounded
with bright eyes and a sweet smile

Chapter 2
Introduction to the Chakra System

Navigating the 7 Major Steps to Healing

There is so much more to you than just your physical body, your biology, the part of you that you can perceive with your five primary senses. Your physical body could not be animated without your life force energy, which is often perceived as sexual energy. Your chakra system is a series of unseen energy centers which correlate to areas of your body and influence many aspects of your being. The energy in your chakras can become blocked or diminished and can begin to manifest imbalances in your body in the form of pain, dis-ease, or illness. If the balance of your energy body can be maintained, the balance of your physical body will follow.

Many bodywork modalities now incorporate "energy work" or "energy healing." Reiki and Healing Touch are two of the most commonly known types of energy healing. Practitioners using this type of modality are channeling universal life force energy through their hands into the chakras of their clients. The universal life force energy balances their energy system and may provide information on a subtle level about problem areas.

The actual responsibility for the healing resides firmly in the client. A practitioner's job is to hold a space for healing and to assist the client in creating the necessary balance within themselves to facilitate healing. In many cases, there are "payoffs" for holding onto a disease or illness, which may be held in the subconscious. More obvious examples would be disability pay or a caretaker lavishing attention, each of which may have to be released along with the illness. It is helpful to have a willingness to probe potentially difficult and painful emotional issues in order to accomplish true healing. Treating the chakras and exploring their associations within the body can be an effective tool for healing of all kinds.

In this book, the chakra system is explored in depth as a healing and recovery journey, a journey from fear to enlightenment. Each chapter focuses on one of the seven major chakras, starting with the base or root chakra, and will incorporate aspects of that chakra's influence on the body, mind, and emotions within the scope of recovery from childhood sexual abuse. Within each chapter are exercises and meditations to help integrate the information into your body through experiential practice. Use this book in whatever way suits you best. Progress through it completely and then start again, working with one chapter at a time; or simply start with the first chapter and work with the exercises at the end before proceeding to the next chapter. You can find bonus guided audios of some of the exercises along with numerous additional resources at amritagrace.com/reclaim.

Chapter 3
First Chakra -The Root of the Issues

Your first chakra, also known as your base or root chakra, is located below the base of your spine in your perineum area. Your first chakra rules your lower pelvic organs and tissues and your rectum, and is considered the foundation of your life: stability, survival, and grounding. The issues that relate to your root chakra are money, home, family, health, structure, work, and security. The color associated with this chakra is red, and its challenging aspect is fear. When you live only in your first chakra, you simply react to life. Your adrenals pump adrenaline and your fight, flee, or freeze response is triggered. There is no logic or thought. The words and actions of others trigger old belief systems and automatic responses. Decisions are fear-based and history-based.

With a healthy first chakra, you are firmly anchored to the earth and grounded in the present moment. There are no worries about the future or your security, because you trust that what you need will be there when you need it. You are comfortable in your home and have a healthy relationship with your family. You enjoy your livelihood and feel that you are doing worthwhile service for others while taking care of yourself and your family. You are in good health and have done whatever you can to insure your healthy future. You understand that living in fear draws to you that which you fear and you work through and process your fears, seeking help when needed.

How Your History Affects You

As a survivor of childhood molestation and abuse, my boundaries were violated in many ways. I was threatened never to tell what was happening to me. Those who were supposed to protect and nurture me were either behaving inappropriately or, in the case of my mother, unable to see what was happening to me right before their eyes. I acquired numerous survival skills from these experiences that carried well into my adulthood and my adult relationships. I unconsciously drew people to me who would help me re-create my childhood experiences, in the hopes of finally resolving the issues. As long as I was unaware of this, the issues were never resolved. I simply replayed the painful circumstances of my childhood over and over, without resolution, in the context of my adult relationships.

When you begin to unravel your buried issues, layer by layer you must acknowledge the feelings associated with them. Instead of keeping the pain buried, where it will drive you unconsciously, you have an opportunity to let it surface and finally be released. The only way *out* is *through*!

Desperation and Denial

As a wounded child living in an adult body, you are driven by desperation to keep the pain of your past experiences deeply buried. Everything you do is a means to this end. The desperation leads to denial of what is right in front of you. By refusing to look at the truth, you maintain the status quo of your tightly bound and controlled world.

My favorite example of denial in my own life went on for almost 15 years. I left my first husband (who kept a messy house) for my second husband in an unconscious act of sexual addiction. I came to the conclusion that my second husband was a very tidy person, because that is what I wanted to see. In reality, I did all the cleaning, because that was one of my compulsions. When we had been separated for a year, our property sold and I went to help clean up before the close of escrow. I volunteered to clean the house while he worked on the garage. What I found in his house was one of the filthiest and most disgusting living situations I have ever seen. I gritted my teeth and did the job I had agreed to do, cleaning up after him one last time. It was quite a lesson in denial for me and I still smile over the irony of it.

Running Away

When the going gets tough, the wounded person runs. Although you may not always run away from your primary relationship, you may run towards some kind of addictive behavior as a way to soothe a painful or difficult period in your primary relationship. Or, you may simply run from one relationship to another in an attempt to find happiness. What you are really running away from is your hurt and pain. Fear is the driving force that keeps you in motion, because if you stop, all that you are running from just might catch up. You may find yourself in the same situations over and over with different people, feeling victimized by circumstances. Eventually, if you are lucky, you begin to see patterns repeat themselves and you can take steps toward making new choices.

Objectifying Others

When you are used as the object of other people's needs as a child, you are given the impression that this is normal behavior for adults. When you are not treated with compassion, you do not learn how to be compassionate. This combination of objectification and lack of compassion can lead you to judge others in a cold and heartless manner. As an adult, I objectified other people the same way I was objectified as a child. I would generally put people in two categories based on how they looked: "potential sex partners" or "not potential sex partners."

The following story is an excellent example of the objectification of a child. Unbeknownst to my mother, I had already lived through several years of sexual and emotional abuse. Although my abuser was no longer in the picture, the damage was done. In this story, you will learn my childhood nickname.

Personal Story: *Judgement Day*

"Janie darling, do you need some lotion for your knees and elbows?" I hear a mother say to her daughter, who is probably all of seven years old. The words float through my mind as I stand in line to be judged. My palms are sweaty under the white gloves that my mom says I have to wear in this stupid pageant. I don't understand why she makes me keep doing this; I am not exactly what you would call pretty. In fact, I am downright ugly.

Cyndi won the first pageant she was in. She has always been the beautiful sister, the favored one. She has all the friends, the good grades, and people are always telling her she should be a model. What I don't understand is why people say we look like twins. How can that be if she is pretty and I am ugly? At least I don't have to compete against her in this pageant. *That* is a losing battle.

My stomach is churning as I approach the steps to the runway. I am trying to remember everything Mom taught me about how to walk and pose. Are my hands right? I think I'm supposed to stick my pinkies out. Oh, yeah, and stand up straight. STAND UP STRAIGHT, STAND UP STRAIGHT, I'm so sick of hearing that. My turn now. I guess I need to paste on a fake smile, because I don't feel like smiling at all right now. I am so embarrassed. What the hell is an ugly duckling like me doing in a beauty pageant anyway?

Oh, my God, they're looking at me like I'm a chicken hanging from a meat hook. Everyone is looking at me! Leave me alone! I just want to hide in my room and be left alone. What can you possibly see that you like, you stupid people? Just an ugly girl in ugly clothes. This runway is endless. I can't believe I have to do this again in a bathing suit.

What a humiliating day. The makeup is hurting my eyes and I keep smearing my lipstick so that I look like a clown. At least I have my friend Karen; she is such a happy person that you can't be sad around her. "Kimmy, it's time for the judges to announce their decision, come on Honey!" I go with Mom to listen to the judgement. The second runner up is announced, and everyone cheers. The first runner up is Karen, and she looks happy and disappointed at the same time. I can't believe she did not win, she is so pretty! The winner is announced and I can't believe my ears. They have said my name. There must be some mistake. Mom pushes me out towards the steps to the runway while simultaneously hugging me.

I am in shock. It can't be true. A smiling judge is handing me a gigantic trophy and pinning a ribbon on my dress that says "Pre-Teen Miss Fresno." The trophy is placed at my side and I feel a little shove towards the runway. This isn't right, Karen is supposed to win! I walk down the runway, and to my horror, I begin to cry. I get all red and blotchy when I cry. Now they'll know for sure they made a mistake. I walk like a frozen mummy. I am numb. I do my best to smile. The flash of a camera blinds me for a moment.

Suddenly I understand. They felt sorry for me! That's why I won! This is my third pageant, and they are sick of me and just want me to go away. Relief floods through me, and the numbness eases. I feel better now and finish my runway walk. I don't have to do this anymore. It's all over.

~

Clearly, it's not all over! This story took place at the approximate age of eleven. It is interesting to note that I only found peace when I came back to a negative view of myself. The situation was exacerbated by the fact that my mother thought we were such beautiful girls and took so much pride in our participation in the pageants. When I look at the photos and remember, I see a young woman lost in the darkness infusing her soul.

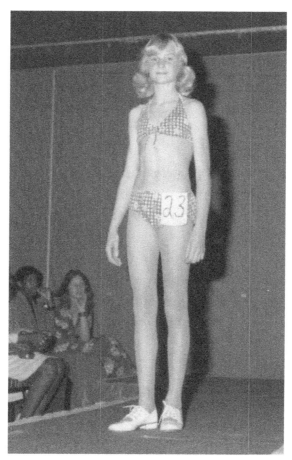

On the runway for the
pre-teen Miss Fresno pageant.

Do You Need Professional Help?

There is a fierce sense of independence that comes with being a survivor. Unwilling to trust anyone else or to be vulnerable in any way, you determine that you can do it all yourself. You place a firm protection around your heart and present yourself as an indestructible fortress. Reaching out for help means breaching the fortress and finding a way to trust others for assistance and support.

Connecting with others who are on a similar path is an acknowledgement that you are not alone and a big step on the path to recovery. You can learn so much from others who are having similar struggles and experiences. Compassion begins to penetrate the cracks in your armor when you see others revealing their pain and vulnerability, sending light into the dark places in your fortress. Trying to recover alone is the hard way and the long way. Having a non-judgmental support system can help you learn compassion and loving kindness for yourself. 12-step programs have helped many people over the years, and yet they are not the answer for everyone. Rational Recovery is another option, as is individual or group therapy.

In the beginning, I worked my own recovery path through a spiritual path. I was also receiving couple's counseling for my marriage issues. I shied away from 12-step programs, unable to find one that met my needs. I found that many therapists did not understand the problem of sexual addiction in women. Several therapists went so far as to dismiss my self-diagnosis of sexual addiction. I was living in a small town in the mountains of California in the late 1990's, and finding no promising resources for myself, I simply did the best I could on my own.

There is a much broader understanding today of sexual addiction issues. Sex Addicts Anonymous is very helpful in that it provides tools for defining sexual sobriety as well as the support of people on the same healing path. I finally made it to some SAA meetings in my eighth year of recovery. While I still find that some of the 12 steps do not resonate with my concepts of personal power and responsibility, I do see the value that others have received from attending meetings, having a sponsor, and sponsoring others. Individual therapy is certainly an option and combines well with other therapies. I recommend locating a therapist who specializes in or is at least well-versed in sexual addiction. If you are a woman with sexual abuse or addiction issues, your treatment needs will be different from a man's treatment needs.

Survival Skills

In cases of sexual molestation, imbalance in the first chakra is characterized by a survival skill often learned at a very young age: leaving the body. This translates to leaving the present moment so that you do not have to experience what is happening in your body, also known as dissociation. As a survival skill, it is very effective; however, it often becomes a habit that continues to be used long after it loses its ability to serve you.

One of my main survival skills was control. Having been controlled as a child, I decided that I was never going to let anyone control me again. By manipulating everything and everyone around me, I created an illusion of perfection and order. I gained a false sense of security that kept me firmly anchored in my first chakra. Perfectionism and extreme rigidity were necessary to keep the illusion of control in place. Over and over, I unconsciously replayed my childhood abuse, putting myself in the place of the aggressor, the one who calls the shots.

Denial is a survival skill as well. Refusing to see anything that will upset the delicate balance of your fragile world is a way of keeping the pain at bay. It's amazing how your mind can construct your reality in keeping with your beliefs.

Exercise 1-1: B-R-E-A-T-H-I-N-G!

You probably don't give much thought or notice to your breathing. It's simply an involuntary bodily function, right? In fact, attention to the breath is a key to your healing process. Deeply breathing moves energy and expands your internal reality. Shallow breathing contracts you and can shut you down. Begin by putting a hand on your belly and pushing your hand out with your inhalation, belly and chest filling fully and emptying completely. Continue this practice for two minutes. Begin a daily practice and add two minutes each week until you find yourself aware of breathing more fully and deeply throughout your daily life.

Exercise 1-2: Getting and Staying Grounded
(bonus audio at amritagrace.com/reclaim)

Create a time in your day when you will not be disturbed for ten minutes to half an hour. Make sure that your phone will not interrupt you. Find a comfortable place to sit where your back is supported and your feet are on the floor. Close your eyes and imagine that you are becoming a tree. As a tree, you are sending roots down into the ground and finding stability within the earth. Feel the roots extending from your feet and sense the energy and support that you draw up through your root system. As a tree, you also have branches and leaves that reach up and out. You take in sunlight and energy from above through your leaves and branches. Feel the energy coming in from above and how it moves down your trunk into your roots. Feel how firmly you are connected to the Earth and anchored in your body. With practice, you can recall this feeling anytime you need to get grounded, sending your energy into your roots to instantly ground yourself.

Exercise 1-3: Keeping a Recovery Journal

Keeping a journal is a wonderful way to review your progress through your healing journey. You can write by hand or on your computer, whatever feels most comfortable to you. Set aside time each day to record whatever you are thinking and feeling. Don't worry about whether it is "presentable" or not, this is only for you. As you take steps toward wholeness and sexual sobriety, you may eventually want to see how far you have come by looking back in your journal. A journal is also an excellent way to discharge your feelings and emotions, effectively moving the energy up and out of you.

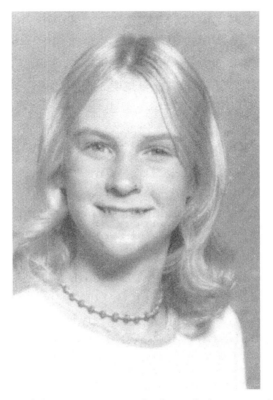

Age thirteen, wounded and damaged...
but nobody knew it yet.

Chapter 4
Second Chakra - Sexual Maturity

Your second chakra, also known as your sacral chakra, is located in your genitals. Many energy work facilitators teach that this chakra is located above your genitals and below your navel, this being a more polite area to touch. Your second chakra rules your reproductive organs, hips, and lower back. The issues that relate to your second chakra are emotions, creativity, and sexuality. The color associated with this chakra is orange, and its difficult aspect is guilt.

When you live only in your second chakra, your emotions and impulses are in control. Hedonism is the doctrine that you live by. You take what you want without heart or thought for anyone else. You do what you want whether it is good for you or not, regardless of whether it's detrimental to you or to others. Your emotions run rampant and may cause damage to others or to yourself. Your relationships with others, whether at work or at home, may involve power struggles and abuse. When observing other people's body language, notice when they protect their second chakra by crossing their legs or by some other action that shields the area. Notice how often you protect this area as well, especially in tense situations.

With a healthy second chakra, you are in the flow of life. You are willing to process through a wide range of emotions, on a continuum from very difficult to extremely joyful. You are able to express your emotions in appropriate ways. Your ethics and morals in dealing with others are sound, and you don't feel a need to have power over others or allow others to have power over you. You are comfortable with your body and your sexuality and make healthy choices in sexual partnerships. You allow time and space for creativity in your life as a form of self-expression. In difficult or tense situations, you are able to stay self-contained and have clear boundaries.

Getting "Switched On"

As I look back over my early adult years, I see my first sexual encounter as an adult as a turning point. It feels to me as if my addiction was "switched on," and I gained a new way to use my power. I went to a whole new level of lying and sneaking around after that first time, and I no longer had any moral compunction to wait "until I was married." Over the next few years, behavior patterns began to emerge that repeated themselves over and over. One of the patterns was feeling attracted to others while I was in a committed relationship. In the beginning, I would end the relationship I was in before getting involved with the object of my attraction. Eventually I would act on the attraction while still involved in a relationship. I left many broken hearts and a trail of emotional devastation in my wake.

The Many Faces of Acting Out: Substituting Addictions

Have you ever noticed how people who quit smoking tend to put on weight? This is a classic example of substituting one addiction for another. Addicts of all kinds have many ways to keep the pain at bay, and multiple addictions are often present. In my first marriage, I only acted out sexually one time in seven years. However, it was with this

28

partner that I became a severe drug abuser. Although I had experimented with various drugs before meeting him, it was with him that I learned to become a regular user. Eventually, I became tired of the lifestyle I was living and began to leave the drugs behind. As I moved away from the drug use, my sexual addiction stepped back in to protect me from my pain and I embarked on an affair with a man I worked with. There was a very intense attraction between us, and although we were both married, we decided we had to be together. I took a week away from my husband to decide what to do, and the following story describes the manner in which I ended my marriage.

Personal Story: *Without Looking Back*

I approach the parking lot for my apartment building filled with trepidation. I park the car and sit there, trying to draw courage into my body by breathing deeply. A late November rain is falling, and the inside of the car gets more steamy and oppressive with every passing second. I can smell the unmistakable scent of my own fear. A memory of my recent birthday drifts through my mind, of how proud I was to be turning a quarter of a century old. I snap myself back to the present, and I know that in the next few minutes, my life is going to change forever.

I walk in the door after being gone for a week, and see my husband Dave sitting on the couch. He gets up to hug me, concern etched across his face. "Are you okay, Honey?" he asks. "There's something I need to talk to you about. Let's sit down," I respond. I begin by trying to break the news as gently as possible. "I can't stay in this relationship anymore, Dave." I see the shock and disbelief on his face. He asks "What are you talking about Kim? We can work through whatever is happening!" "I'm sorry, Dave, I've made my decision." He responds, "Don't I get to have any say in this?" I put my hand on his knee, and with sorrow and regret, I tell him that there is another person involved. "I have been having an affair, and I want to be with him." The shock and disbelief turn to anger, and he says, "You have been cheating on me? How could you violate the sanctity of this marriage, of our vows? I can't believe you would do this to me."

I start to cry. He asks who the man is, and in a gesture of protection, I say only his first name. Everything around me looks surreal. The brown couch, the lamp on the table in the corner, and the ashtray on the coffee table full of cigarette butts seem like articles from another planet. I clearly see that I won't ever live in this apartment again.

"You cheap slut! You ruined our beautiful marriage," I hear him say as if from another dimension. I sense it is time to leave. "I'm going to go stay at my sister's house for a while," I tell him as I get up from the couch. "Wait, Kim, you can't leave me, I love you!" he says, his face now reflecting sadness and fear. "I have to go, Dave," I say as I grab my purse and head for the door.

The late November afternoon has turned into evening. It is still raining. I sit in my car, letting the guilt wash over me for just a moment before I shift my thoughts to Larry, my new love. I take a deep breath and focus on my future as I start the car and head for a new life.

~

Does this scenario feel achingly familiar to you? Have you thrown people away in your life in a similar manner? Substituting one partner for another is very much like substituting addictions. It is a way of leaving the old behind and being stimulated by something fresh and new. It is an excellent way to stay distracted.

Do You Have an Addiction?

The words "sex addict" can conjure up images of flashers in trench coats, of dirty old men hanging around schoolyards, of perverts frequenting the porno theaters. In reality, most people who are acting out sexually are regular people with regular jobs. They have been so badly injured as children that their compulsions have become a way of life. If you are reading this book right now, chances are you want to find a way to free yourself from acting-out behavior, and perhaps your acting-out behavior has been of a sexual nature.

The book *Rational Recovery, The New Cure for Substance Addiction* defines "addiction" as "a chemical dependency that exists against one's own better judgement and persists in spite of efforts to control or eliminate the use of the substance. Logically, since addiction is known only to the individual, it may not be 'diagnosed' except by asking the individual." This brings up two different questions:

- Is sexual addiction a chemical dependency?

- Can a person really be diagnosed by anyone other than himself or herself?

To address the first question, I believe that sexual

31

addiction *is* a chemical dependency. The pleasurable feelings and chemical releases into the bloodstream that accompany sex, fantasizing, masturbation, and other (normally) pleasurable activities have the same effect on a sex addict as heroin has on a drug addict. Those pleasurable feelings offer the same level of escape from pain and discomfort as any other substance. For a sex addict, they are the drug of choice.

The second question focuses on diagnosis, and brings us back to the chapter title: Do you have an addiction? It is my belief that each person must make that assessment for themselves. The following questions may help you better examine your actions and their consequences:

- Do you have feelings of shame or guilt before, during, or after sex?

- Do you feel as though you can't stop yourself from being sexual in some situations?

- Do you coerce or pressure others into being sexual with you?

- Are you easily convinced to have sex, even when you don't really want to?

- Do you use sex with others as a way to punish your partner?

- Do you masturbate when you are upset?

- Do you spend a considerable amount of time fantasizing about sexual encounters?
- Do you lie to anyone about your sex partners?

- Do you put yourself at risk for sexually transmitted diseases or violence?

- Do you spend inordinate amounts of time participating in pornography?

If you answered yes to any of these questions, you may have addiction issues that bear looking at.

Sex and Love Addictions

Sometimes sex and love become so intertwined that it becomes nearly impossible to separate them. If a parent has an incestuous relationship with a child, the child learns that love is given in the form of sexual attention. Later in life, the adult incest survivor may have to contend with an indelible link between being loved and being sexual.

Who Hurt You, Little One?

It has been my experience that sexual addiction stems from sexual abuse. When a child is abused and mistreated by an adult, especially a person the child knows and trusts, the child is left powerless. When a child is threatened not to tell anyone about what happened to him or her, they are left without resources. As the child gets older, opportunities to reclaim his or her power begin to present themselves. Using the behavior that has been learned by example from the abuser, the child may begin to abuse and mistreat others in an unconscious way.

When I meet people either with sex addictions or who are themselves sexual abusers, the first question that comes to mind is "Who hurt you, little one?" I even extend this compassionate approach to my own abuser when I think of him. It took me many years of process to get to that point, however! It is important to acknowledge the anger and find healthy expression for it with regard to those who have hurt you. Forgiveness and compassion will come in time for some, and may not ever come for others.

The "little one" that was hurt continues to live on inside us. I have a seven-year old that resides in my third chakra (solar plexus) area that I call "Little Kim." For many years, she made most of the decisions about my life from her place in my unconscious. She locked up my heart, building a fortress with iron gates around it. She tapped into the power of my adult body and mind, using them to exact her revenge. With her guiding me, I became a sexual predator. I objectified people, overpowered them, attempted to manipulate and control them. Her role was a protective one. As long as she was calling the shots, there was no way that we would be feeling any pain. At the first sign of a painful memory or reminder of the past, she would steer us toward a distraction as quickly as possible. She was especially active in love relationships, where quite often, our partner would hold up a mirror that showed us our pain.

Exercise 2-1: Creating Inner Sanctuary
(bonus audio at amritagrace.com/reclaim)

No matter what is going on around you, you always have

the option of going inside and finding inner sanctuary. Find a quiet place where you can be alone and begin to practice your breathing and grounding exercises. As you sink deeply into relaxation, imagine you are on a forest path, and that the path is leading you to a place of sanctuary where nothing and no one can harm you or disturb you. Take note of what you see there; take in the colors, sounds, scents, textures, and features of this place. It may be a room or building or an outdoor space. Allow your imagination to supply the information.

You will have the opportunity to return to this place over and over. This is your personal inner sanctuary. Create it however you want to, so that you feel cradled and nurtured. As you complete with the visualization, describe your sanctuary in your journal.

Exercise 2-2: Breathing Up To Your Heart
(bonus audio at amritagrace.com/reclaim)

Find a quiet space and go to your inner sanctuary. Find a comfortable place to sit in your sanctuary, and begin to practice your breathing and grounding. Invite your awareness to slowly descend into your second chakra. Now, send your breath all the way down into your second chakra as you inhale. As you exhale, bring your energy and awareness up to your heart. Now breathe your energy back down to your second chakra, and feel the circulation between your heart and your second chakra. Breathe in this manner for as long as you feel comfortable, continuing to keep your focus inside yourself and breathing deeply and slowly.

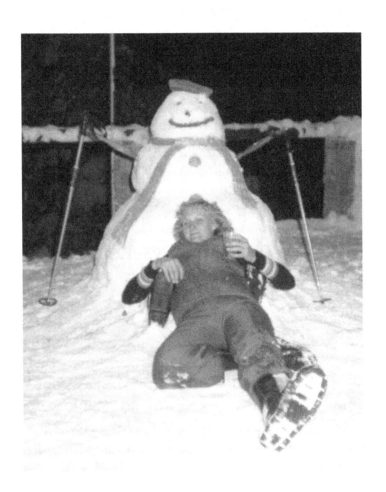

Age eighteen, with alcoholic beverage in hand.
The "sex, drugs, & rock & roll" years.

Chapter 5
Third Chakra – Inner Self: Inner Child

Your third chakra, also known as your solar plexus chakra, is located below your rib cage junction and in your upper belly. Your third chakra rules your stomach, intestinal tract, pancreas, and adrenal glands. The issues that relate to your third chakra are personal power, strength of will, self-mastery, self-esteem, and individuation. The color associated with this chakra is yellow, and its challenging aspect is shame. Your third chakra is the home of your inner child, the place of your identity. When your third chakra is closed, you may attempt to feed your personal power through controlling people and situations in your life.

Wounded children are often dominated and manipulated. In an effort to overcome this feeling, they may strive to dominate and manipulate others. A closed third chakra is like an ivory tower from which you can sit and judge everything around you, which really amounts to judgements about yourself. Acceptance, allowing, and non-attachment are nearly impossible to cultivate from this hiding place.

With a healthy and open third chakra, you are secure in your self-image and have a high degree of self-esteem. You are creating a positive energetic vibration in the world around you because you are comfortable with yourself and confident about what you have to offer the world. You have established a loving, compassionate relationship with your inner child, and you have a continuing inner practice of healthy parenting for him or her. When the needs of your inner child are being met, he or she no longer runs in survival mode with the need to act out for attention.

In the Driver's Seat Without a License

Imagine the metaphor of a six-year old child driving a car. In order to reach the gas pedal, she must slide down on the seat. She presses the gas, and the car speeds off... but she cannot see where she is going because she is too small. She feels the power of the car moving under her and that power fills her up and makes her pain go away. She races through the streets of life, running over whatever is in her way in a chaotic and desperate attempt to be in control of her destiny.

You are the six-year old in this metaphor and the car is your body. Is it any wonder you feel like your life is out of control? The first impulse in a closed third chakra might be to be angry with the child. You may want to make him or her stop at all costs, using the same control and manipulation techniques that he or she has been using without your conscious knowledge. If this is happening, know that it is a perfectly natural part of the process, and that with time and inner work, you can bring loving compassion to your angry and hurting little ones.

The metaphor of the car also corresponds to what you are creating in your life. If you are not consciously creating your life, then you are unconsciously creating it. If you are unable to see over the steering wheel, you are essentially blindly manifesting the circumstances around you. As humans, each of us has the ability to consciously co-create everything that happens in our lives. The little one that has so much power to create chaos also has the same power to create peace and contentment. So how do you go about making the necessary changes? The first step is to get acquainted.

Exercise 3-1: Getting Acquainted
(bonus audio at amritagrace.com/reclaim)

Close your eyes and imagine yourself when you were little. Work with whatever image comes to mind and take note of the age you imagine yourself to be. Imagine yourself with that child, as if she is a separate being, and notice what she seems to be feeling. Is she frightened? Angry? Petrified with fear? Is there anyone she can trust, or does she feel like she is alone and abandoned? Don't be surprised if you can't stay with her for very long just now. Notice how you feel toward her. Do you feel aversion and disgust or compassion and empathy? Most likely at this stage you will feel somewhat repulsed by her as she reveals feelings that you have been pushing away for some time now.

Trusting Your Little Ones

Third chakra healing involves ongoing work with your wounded inner child. As I began this work for myself, I made an important discovery. I knew there was a huge trust issue between myself and Little Kim, but I thought that it was about her not trusting me. What it was really about was me not trusting her. During my recovery work, I put her in a cage so that she would stop acting out, thereby closing up my third chakra and sealing her inside. I was more than seven years into my recovery before I realized what I had done. The cage I created effectively kept Little Kim under control and effectively shut down my third chakra. As I gained an understanding of what I had done, I sought help to begin the process of releasing her and giving her a voice. We'll talk more about your voice when we get to the fifth chakra chapter.

For this work, I found a hypnotherapist who was adept at regression therapy. Through my work with her, I had a huge third chakra opening and gave Little Kim some freedom and room to move. Although I had been doing inner child work off and on for the previous seventeen years, this step moved me into a whole new realm of openness, expansiveness, and compassion. The first thing we did was to get Little Kim out of the cage. Patricia, the hypnotherapist, said, "No one wants to live in a cage." I was stunned by the simplicity of this statement. It had never occurred to me that I had been mistreating my inner child.

Moving Little Kim out of her cage and into another space was a huge step in opening my third chakra. During the session, another amazing thing happened. At the end of the visualization, Little Kim said some words. Again, I was stunned, for it didn't occurred to me that she had never spoken before until I heard her words. The words were, "Let's play!"

In the next hypnotherapy session, we did some regression work with Little Kim. Patricia took me through some various scenarios, giving Little Kim a chance to say whatever she needed to and was unable to say as a little girl. She kept regressing me farther back, until much to the surprise of both of us, I was in the womb! I received tremendous insight from my experience in the womb. I learned that the fetus is full of knowledge and perception. Even more importantly, I learned why becoming invisible was such a comfortable survival technique for me in childhood, a technique that I carried into adulthood.

Personal Story: *Hiding*

I'm not quite sure why yet, but Mom is hiding me. Every day, I am flooded with her shame and guilt. I am a dirty secret that must be kept quiet as long as possible. It's warm and dark in this place, and I haven't many cares...except for Mom's intense feelings that jolt through me in her waking hours.

Weeks pass, and she talks about me in whispers to Aunt Janeen in the bedroom they share. "You mustn't tell Mom and Dad until after our summer vacation," Aunt Janeen urges her. Mom is scared. I can feel it every day.

At night, when Mom is sleeping, I have peace in my dark, watery world. I roll and tumble in the amniotic fluid, enjoying the sensation of being free from worry. If only she could just love me; after all, we chose each other...doesn't she remember?

I can feel that something is different today. Mom has pushed the shame and guilt into the background of her mind, and has replaced it with fierce determination. I think she is going to reveal my presence! I am filled with simple joy over this realization.

"Oh, my God, Sharron, you have ruined your life!" I hear Grandmother wail. Her voice is so loud that I am rocked by waves in the fluids that surround me. The shame and guilt flood me again as they wash over Mother. Grandmother continues to wail and cry. Now Mom is crying too. She is so ashamed of me.

"That boy is going to have to marry you now, you know!" I hear Grandmother say, the register of her voice lowering from anger to shock. I feel Mom's thought, "At least I will get out of this hellhole..."

I'm so glad I am not in hiding anymore! Maybe now we can simply love each other as we are meant to do.

~

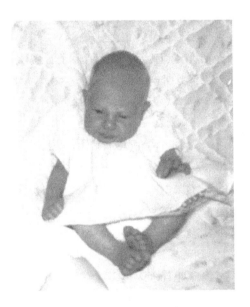

One month old

The Reparenting Process

Once you've met the child that lives on inside of you, it's important to take steps toward having regular contact with her. Most likely she has not had a healthy parental figure influencing her, and you have an opportunity to correct that. You can call upon your own wise inner being or inner mom to reparent your lost little inner kid. The first step is to establish regular contact with him or her. Setting aside a few minutes each day in which to close your eyes and reach out (in) to him or her is a good beginning. In this process, trust and compassion can slowly be built. I recommend starting with a simple healing intention. You can even use a teddy bear or other "stuffy" to represent your inner child, so that whenever you see the bear, you remember to take some time with him or her.

It is helpful to use visualization techniques to create a safe inner sanctuary where you can have contact with your inner child. This place can be a sunny meadow, a hut on the beach, a warm pool, a room with a rocking chair, a classroom, or whatever your imagination and your inner kid wants to create. Most importantly, the space should feel safe and comforting. You can return to this space regularly and spend quality time getting acquainted with and reparenting your inner kid(s).

Nourishing the New Kid

Your inner kid will have individual needs to be attended to, depending on what was missing in your childhood situations. One way to find out what is needed is to ask your little one in a visualization. This process may or may not be successful on the first attempt, and it is important to gently keep trying until your little one has a chance to trust the process and find his or her voice. Patience is the key here, along with willingness and compassion.

Reconnecting with what was missing in your childhood can bring up lots of trauma and pain, as well as feelings of vulnerability, rejection, abandonment, fear, helplessness, anger, grief, and loss. By simply being with these feelings, rather than acting to hide from them, suppress them, or push them away, you have an opportunity to feel them and then release them. Perhaps your pattern in the past has been to "act out," either sexually or in some other way, to keep these feelings at bay. Your opportunity now is to sit with the feelings, experience them, allow them to wash over you, and then to recognize that you have the capacity to process and release each of these feelings.

It's helpful in the process to understand that emotions are like ocean waves. They sneak up, peak, crash, and recede. Sometimes, when you are deep in the grip of an emotion, it seems like it will never end. If you can remember, in that moment, that emotions are like waves, you can remember that they will eventually peak, crash, and recede. You can learn to ride the emotional waves like a skilled surfer.

Acknowledging the feelings that have kept you bound is a huge step toward freedom, and it does get easier with practice. If it all feels just too overwhelming, it is possible to break this process down into smaller pieces and work with one emotion at a time. In my own process, I found that I had a tremendous amount of stored grief. I realized that I had gone straight from one love relationship to another, without a break, for my entire adult life, never grieving the loss of the previous partner. One day I simply decided it was time to feel all my grief, and for the next eight months, people and situations steadily showed up to help me do just that. The following story illustrates one of the events that took place to help me grieve.

Personal Story: *Ghosts with Unusual Names*

I saw a new patient tonight at the chiropractor's office where I work as a massage therapist. His name was Chet, and he was very sweet. He told me his fiancé would be meeting him after the massage since it's walking distance from her job. As I left the massage room to let Chet get dressed, I encountered a roomful of people in the lobby. I looked in the calendar to see who my next patient was as Chet came out of the room looking relaxed. He wove through the crowded room to make his next appointment with me. He asked, "Have you met my fiancé?" "No, I haven't," I answered, and he reached his hand out to her and pulled her from the chair. I said hello and introduced myself to her. She said, "My name is Sundara," and I replied, "Wow, I used to know a little girl named Sundara. How old are you?" "28," she replied. "What is your dad's name?" I asked, and she said Joe. I shook my head as if trying to clear the cobwebs of many years. "What is your mom's name?" I asked. She said exactly what I expected her to say, "Julie." I asked, "And your mom is gone now?" "Yes," she replied. "I used to babysit you when you were a little girl!" I exclaimed.

My mind was reeling. Chet was interested in the conversation, but also looking at me expectantly to schedule his next appointment. People in the waiting room had stopped talking and were listening to our exchange. I felt blood pounding in my ears and the room grew dim as I tried to comprehend the fact that a ghost from my past had appeared in my midst. If it weren't for her unusual name, I never would have recognized her. My next patient was waiting and I had to find a way to function. I couldn't let the dammed-up memories break through just yet, because I might drown if they came too fast. Taking a deep breath, I got Chet scheduled, asked Sundara for her phone number, and made my way back into the massage room to change the sheets.

Once I had the next patient on the table, I let my body take over and allowed the flood of memories to wash over me. I was momentarily amazed that I could calmly go through the motions of massage while my mind was exploding with intensity. The first two things to hit me were the manner of Julie's death and the manner in which I was told about Julie's death.

Julie was Sundara's mom, and she was part of a group of friends I had when I was married to my first husband, Dave. I left her and all my other friends behind when I left Dave for Larry. About 4 years into my marriage to Larry, I came home from work to a written message by the phone. It said, "Patty called, Julie died, hung herself, Brad found her." Ouch. What a way to learn of an old friend's suicide! I was not invited to her funeral, nor would I have gone. That would mean facing my shame over the husband and friends that I threw away. I was sure they would not want me there.

Memories continued to tumble through my mind. I got a visual on a huge box of photos in a closet in my apartment, and I began to anticipate getting home and going through that box. I would find pictures of Julie to give to Sundara and that would be a way to connect with her.

As I brought the heavy box down from a high shelf, I had a sense of what Pandora must have felt like before she opened her box. Nothing was ever going to be the same again once the top came off. As I sorted through hundreds of pictures of another life, I came to an understanding. Sundara was an angel of mercy, sent to help me do exactly what I asked for—to grieve all that I have not yet grieved. I laughed and cried, and I marveled at the love and happiness I saw on my face in the photos. I set aside the photos of Julie for Sundara and began a pile for Dave. We hadn't spoken in at least fifteen years, but I knew his address.

I kept a small pile of photos for myself and put them in an envelope. I boxed up the stack for Dave and sent them off to him. I would have loved to burn the rest, but I couldn't figure out how to do that appropriately in my Oakland apartment building. Putting them into three full brown grocery bags, I blessed them and took them out to the trash.

Two months later, I got a letter from Dave. He and his family were enjoying the photos. He talked about his many recent experiences of things coming full circle. He wrote, "And so you know, I have had to forgive you for what you did to our lives, quite a while ago. It didn't hurt you for me to be mad, it only hurt me. There is a little gremlin that pokes his head up every now and then, but I have released the past, so you can too." He signed the letter with a peace symbol and signed it Love, Dave.

For the first time in seventeen years, I had made peace with this piece of my past. I give thanks for angels of mercy and ghosts with unusual names.

~

In some cases, the feelings cannot be separated and felt individually because they are so intertwined. Abandonment and rejection are often closely tied together and are not actually feelings as such, but are indicators of feelings underneath them. Shame and guilt are emotions that are often linked. You must trust that what is offered for you to experience is never going to be more than you are capable of handling. As you untangle the web of old emotions, you create a space for newfound clarity in your life. You gain new perspectives on yourself, on other people, and on the situations you encounter. You become better equipped to make decisions that are in your own best interests.

Exercise 3-2: Integrating Adult, Child, and Infant
(bonus audio at amritagrace.com/reclaim)

For this meditation, make sure you will be undisturbed for at least twenty minutes. Sit in a comfortable position, close your eyes, and go to your sanctuary. Find a place to get comfortable there. When you feel ready, allow an infant to appear next to you. Pick her up and notice how you feel about her. Look at her and really see her (or feel her if you are not getting a visual image). What color are her eyes? What is she wearing? Is she content or agitated? Hold her and send her your love until you feel connected and bonded with her. Next, allow a young child to appear next to you. Let her sit down and then put the baby in her arms. Notice how she reacts to the baby, and the baby to her. Send them both your love, and when the time feels right, invite the little child to absorb the baby into her chest area. Take the child upon your lap and hold her in your embrace. Send her love until you feel connected and bonded, and then allow her to be absorbed into your chest area. Wrap your arms around yourself and feel the integration of your baby and child selves into your adult self. When you feel ready, open your eyes and record your experience in your recovery journal.

Exercise 3-3: Learning to Play

For most wounded children, playing was not a top priority. A difficult home life may have kept you busy learning and implementing your survival skills. One of my own survival skills was to become ultra-responsible. I was the oldest child, my parents worked, and I had siblings that were much younger. I was given lots of responsibility and expected to complete all chores before I was allowed to play. I continued to carry the concept that *all the work must be done before I can play*, even as an adult. I still consciously carve out special time to play in my life, because in truth, the work is never, ever done!

Check in with your inner child, asking her what she likes to do for play. If she doesn't know, you might suggest clay, painting, or drawing. Does she prefer to play alone or with others? Make a special trip to get supplies for the new play activities. Set aside several hours for the first "play date" with your inner child. Don't worry about being messy or how or when to clean up. Let your responsible adult self fall away as you create just for the sake of creating. Whatever you make does not need to be pretty or even

49

presentable. It only needs to be fun. Notice how it feels to play without an agenda. Record your thoughts in your recovery journal.

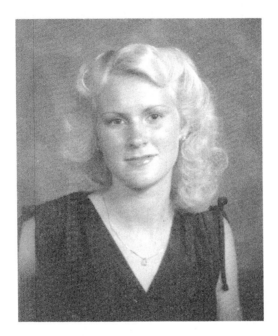

Senior photo, circa 1979

Chapter 6
Fourth Chakra - Heart Opening

The fourth chakra, also known as the heart center, is located in the center of your chest over your heart and lungs. It influences those organs along with your thymus gland. The fourth chakra is connected to love in all its forms: self-love, romantic love, unconditional love, and familial love. The color associated with this chakra is green, and its difficult aspect is grief. Compassion, gratitude, and forgiveness are also closely connected to the fourth chakra. When the fourth chakra is closed, you can become a harsh and critical judge of others and of yourself. An inability to love yourself may stem from past hurts and a need to protect yourself from the perceived threat of future pain. This perceived threat might lead to emotional armoring in an effort to keep your heart "safe." With a closed heart chakra, you limit your ability to fully engage in intimate and familial relationships and friendships.

With a healthy and open fourth chakra, you care for and nurture yourself first and foremost, knowing that if you are able to fully love yourself, you can then fully love others. You are able to recognize the higher being in others no matter what they look like or how they are acting. You can have compassion for others without needing to take on or try to fix their problems or change them. You have strong and well-placed boundaries and you recognize that we each create the reality that we are living in. You are able to love unconditionally, without attachment to outcomes. You are present in each moment, without the need to spin out future fantasies or rehash the past. You freely express your gratitude for all that you have created for yourself, including the difficult lessons. You are able to give and receive without the need to keep score.

Unlocking the Iron Gates

I experienced my own closed fourth chakra as my heart being locked behind iron gates. The iron gates were my armoring, my protection from any potential pain. Little Kim was the keeper of the gates. I was not aware of any of this until I became willing to begin looking at the pain that I previously avoided at all costs. The cost of keeping the pain at bay was actually much higher. I was unable to share myself in relationships and had no concept of intimacy. My behaviors were largely unconscious and were designed to insulate me from my childhood wounding as well as protect me from any pain that might present itself. Paradoxically, over and over, I unconsciously re-created relationships in which I replayed out my childhood circumstances in a largely unsuccessful effort to heal them.

It's helpful to notice the way in which you occupy your body. Is your posture upright, leading with your heart; or do you protect your heart chakra by slouching and rounding your shoulders forward? How often do you cross your arms over your chest in an unconscious effort to reinforce the iron gates? Do you literally turn your back on people or situations that might breach your internal security? Noticing your body language gives you information about the ways in which you protect yourself automatically.

Unlocking the iron gates involves a committed willingness

to become vulnerable and to experience the layers of pain that you have stuffed into your body and your energy field. Because you have spent a lifetime denying the emotions that have closed your heart chakra, it will take some time and patience to peel away the layers. In the beginning, it's helpful to have coaching and guidance in this process. Some people do better with individual counseling or therapy, and others receive more benefit from group situations or more accelerated processes.

In my own journey, I first began to unlock the iron gates in a Landmark Forum-style transformational training workshop. I was five years into my recovery and had recently left my marriage of fourteen years. I was ready for an accelerated, experiential group process and I was not disappointed. In this type of workshop, well-designed activities are given which allow one to look at how they behave in certain situations. Once the behavior is exposed, a choice can be made about whether it is aligned with their current values and whether or not it serves those values. Transformational work such as this can be a way for you to deeply connect with yourself and others on an accelerated track. It has been my experience that I begin these types of workshops with strangers and leave them with family members.

There are many kinds of transformational workshops being offered. Some are more spiritual and some, like the one I experienced, are quite secular. Other organizations offer transformational workshops on love, intimacy, and sexuality. Transformational trainings are for those who are ready to move at an accelerated rate and have lots of breakthroughs in a short space of time. Workshops held exclusively for women are offered in the form of Divine

Feminine workshops, women's retreats, goddess retreats, and my own Sacred Feminine Mystery School's Sacred Sexual Awakening and Healing (AH)™ workshops and certification trainings for women.

Self-Acceptance

One of the biggest keys to unlocking your heart is cultivating the ability to accept yourself just as you are, right now. Self-acceptance dissolves the constant need to judge yourself as not good enough and always needing improvement. At times, this may feel like a paradox. Of course, we all want to become whole, healthy people, and that takes a commitment to work on ourselves. However, if you can simply accept yourself and release the resistance to the parts of yourself you don't like, you can begin to know a glimmer of peace.

Part of self-acceptance is the acceptance all of who you are, even those parts you consider to be ugly or unlikable. You can shed the light of compassion on your whole being, integrating all of your parts into wholeness. Your willingness to embrace all of who you are creates more tolerance for all beings, with their shadows and all. Looking at your inner dark places is never easy, but it is very worthwhile. And, like all the rest of this work, it's a process. A helpful part of this process of acknowledging your darkness can begin with allowing space in your life for sadness, grieving, and times of darkness.

In the Sumerian myth of the descent of Inanna, we learn the story of the underworld journey. The story begins with Inanna wishing to go to the Underworld. She decks herself out in all her royal regalia and proceeds to the gates. She instructs her servant woman what to do if she does not return. She proceeds to the first gatekeeper, who is not impressed. He goes to the Queen of the Underworld, Ereshkigal, who is Inanna's sister. Ereshkigal is not too happy with this intrusion. She tells the gatekeeper to deliver Inanna to her, stripped and in a crouched position. This, by the way, is the way the ancients were buried, stripped and crouching, so Inanna is to be delivered as one dead. At each of the seven gates to the Underworld, Inanna is commanded to strip away some part of her regalia until she is naked. Once in the presence of Ereshkigal, Inanna makes the intention of her visit known, as she removes her sister from the throne and sits in her place. But the powerful Anunnaki gods do not look kindly upon Inanna's attempt and, being the seven Judges of Hades, judge her and condemn her to death. She is killed and hung on a meat hook on the wall. All this time, her servant woman awaits her return. After three days, she realizes that Inanna is not returning, and the servant goes to Anu and pleads for Inanna, asking that Inanna be treated as the Goddess she really is, not as a mortal. Anu, however, is not willing to go against Ereshkigal, saying, "The underworld is for Ereshkigal and Ereshkigal is for the underworld." The woman servant then goes to Ellil, who is just as reluctant. She then goes to Enki, and he has an idea. He fashions two mourners from spit and mud and sends them to Ereshkigal. He also gives each the mourners the water of life and the grass of life to use on Inanna. The two mourners are taken to Ereshkigal, and her vanity gets the better of her as she is offered this attention. When she is not looking, the figures throw the grass of life and the water of life on Inanna and she is returned to original form. She is about to ascend from the Underworld when the Anunnaki gods again interpose. She must appoint a substitute to take her place. She is to return to the Overworld and send a replacement. She encounters her woman servant. She does not send her, though, for what payment is that for such loyalty? She then encounters her husband, Dumuzi, whom she agrees to send. But her husband's sister, Geshtinanna, the wine goddess, intervenes, offering herself instead. The agreement is reached that Dumuzi is to be sent to the Underworld for half a year and his sister is to take his place for the other half of the year.

What this myth symbolizes is the cycle of living and dying; of sadness and happiness; of good times and difficult times; and of light and dark in the seasonal circling of the earth around the sun. What you can glean from this myth is the appropriateness of these natural cycles. Sometimes you feel good, sometimes you feel lousy. Perhaps when you feel down, you beat yourself up or decide you are "bad" or "wrong." With compassion at the helm, a journey to the underworld can be full of revelations. When you accept and support yourself through times of feeling out-of-sorts, chances are you will be able to gain clarity from the chaos. The underworld is a natural place in the cycle of life. Now, when I am feeling lousy about life, I simply acknowledge to myself that I am in the underworld, and sit with whatever is revealing itself to me during that time.

Releasing Control

When you're emotionally shut down, you feel the need to exert a great deal of control over your circumstances and situations. This can be an exhausting illusion to maintain. Imagine what a relief it will be to not have to hold yourself responsible for that which you have no influence over.

When control is surrendered, trust and faith take its place. A space is created for the knowingness that everything that is needed will show up in the perfect time and place. By releasing control, you also release your tendency to set yourself up for failure and disappointment. You release your attachments to a specific outcome, opening the way for infinite possibilities.

The twin sister of control is perfectionism. When you must do everything yourself because no one will do it as well as you do, you are immersed in your control issues. When you have zero tolerance for any kind of messiness or chaos, physical, emotional, mental or otherwise, your control issues have you by the throat. Releasing control is a process that takes time to relax into. It's a process of allowing others to be who they are without needing to manipulate them, and allowing yourself to be who you are without needing to prove anything to yourself or anyone else.

Accessing Vulnerability

The concept of vulnerability is sometimes misconstrued as being a doormat or having an absence of good boundaries. On the contrary, vulnerability can be a place of strength and power and comes from a place of love rather than fear. There is an unshakable aura of self-confidence that is present in a person who is willing to be vulnerable. In order to be vulnerable, you must be willing to drop masks and walls and show up with your true feelings, even if you don't "look good" as a result. Perhaps you're feeling sad or grieving. Instead of pretending to be strong and appearing stoic, you share with others that you are sad. You sit with your feelings instead of covering them up. When you're vulnerable, you can receive support from others without being a victim or a martyr. By showing up with your true feelings, you show others that they can trust you and take you at face value.

It can be rather scary in the beginning to show up vulnerable. For myself, I began to experience true vulnerability when I finally allowed Little Kim to reveal herself through me. I was in my early forties when I finally felt safe enough in my own body to allow this on a regular basis. There were a number of circumstances that brought this situation into reality for me, but mainly it was a realization that I could not proceed any further until I could let this little, unloved part of myself to be seen and heard.

Little Kim, acting through my unconscious, began to project more and more dramatic re-creations of my childhood until I could no longer ignore her. When these dramas would take place, I would show up as a six-year old in an adult body with an adult voice. Already eight plus years into sexual addiction recovery, and with sexual acting-out behavior well behind me, the dramas manifested as behavioral aspects that had been unaddressed during my addiction recovery years.

The pattern that kept repeating went something like this: I would find myself in a community situation, usually a festival or gathering, and there was lots of work that needed to be done to make sure that everyone was comfortable. I would easily slip into "worker drone" mode, a safe and comfortable childhood pattern and a way of avoiding feelings. The controlling perfectionist would step in, work constantly without rest or play, and become very critical and judgmental of everyone else present because they were not working hard enough. In a situation that could have been joyful service with the help and cooperation of a community, I would become isolated and resentful, depriving myself of any fun or play. This repeating situation finally happened in such a dramatic way that it could no longer be ignored. For several weeks after the event, I was exhibiting signs of depression. I thought I would recover, but I did not. I was spiraling downward and my vitality was seeping away from me. Pain was manifesting in my lower back and hip. I was constantly on the verge of tears. Little Kim was no longer going to hide. A dear friend came to my rescue by telling me I had to face whatever what going on inside or I was going to go down hard. I took his advice, looked deeply inside myself, and was able to see the pattern that had re-emerged. Only then could I address the underlying issue. Once addressed, the pattern has never repeated itself again.

Loving Unconditionally

When you love unconditionally, it doesn't matter what others say or do. You have no preconceived notion of how they should act. You do not project your own issues onto them. You simply love them for exactly who they are, in this moment, without expectations or attachments. It doesn't matter if they return the love. It's likely that the most difficult person to love unconditionally is your own self. Most people tend to judge themselves more harshly than they judge others, setting up conditions and expectations.

An amazing thing happens when you find the capacity to

love yourself unconditionally: you find a wellspring of compassion for yourself and others. When compassion rules your heart, the inner critic seems to lose her voice. She may try to speak up and cut you down, but your compassion for yourself overrules her with... more compassion! Your critic responds to this loving support and seems to soften her previously harsh and demanding presence.

Another amazing thing happens when you are able to love yourself unconditionally: you access your ability to embody the divine part of yourself that is inherent in your being. If you choose to take this path, you can call upon this divine part of yourself to be fully present in your body during a sacred ritual or ceremony. My own experience of this process manifested with my first ever sacred, ritualized encounter with a male sexual healing practitioner. During our session, he embodied the energy of Shiva (the archetypal masculine life force energy), which allowed me to naturally embody Shakti (Shiva's counterpart, the archetypal feminine life force energy), taking our connection to a totally transpersonal (beyond personality) level. What I noticed from this experience is that I was in the present moment the whole time. I didn't think of anything else until I sat up and looked around after the session, at which time I realized that I had not left the present moment the entire time. This was a brand new experience for me.

Exercise 4-1: Forgiving Yourself

As you begin to take responsibility for all that you have created in your life, your perceived wrongs may become painful burdens that you carry with you. You have an opportunity to relieve yourself of those burdens by discharging and releasing them. Begin by writing down on paper every single thing you can think of that you perceive you have done wrong. Unburden your soul in as much detail as you need to. As you do so, notice how you feel. Perhaps you feel discomfort. There may be a strong sense of relief. Continue this process until you have discharged everything you feel shameful or guilty about that has transpired in the past.

Next, you are going to forgive yourself for all the things you have written down. While looking in the mirror and holding the paper, speak out loud to yourself, saying something like, "I forgive you for all the past wrongs you have done. I acknowledge you for your courage in taking responsibility. I honor you for your commitment to move forward in integrity." Let these words really reach you to the core of your being.

Now burn the paper, allowing it to be released fully from you. Notice how you feel as you let the paper burn. This process can be cleansing, clearing, and transforming.

Exercise 4-2: Receiving

Learning to receive can be very difficult for those who have struggled with self-esteem issues and control issues. Keeping score can be a survival technique, a way to make sure that you are not in anyone's debt. It can also be a very restrictive behavior. In learning to receive, you must sometimes ask for what you want or need from another. Once you've asked and your request has been agreed to, you must surrender fully to receiving. Learning to ask for what you want and need is a key to this exercise.

For the Receiving exercise, think about something that you would like to receive from another person. For example, you may want to be taken out to dinner by your spouse, or receive a massage after a hard day of work. Perhaps you have hinted around for something in the hopes that you would not have to ask for it outright. For purposes of this exercise, it's important to ask for something from someone. This is not a negotiation of give and take or a trade, but something you are asking for and will not be reciprocating. Does it feel uncomfortable yet? This is a stretch for most of us, because as humans, we are hardwired to reciprocate.

Once you've made an agreement with someone to receive from, you have an opportunity to fully surrender. You may experience feelings of guilt, shame, or remorse for not "contributing your share." Allow these feelings to be felt and wash over you (ride the wave). Thank the feelings for the information and release them with compassion. Receive with gratitude and joy. Express your appreciation graciously. Know that you deserve to be given to. Know that are worthy of the abundance that comes from fully receiving.

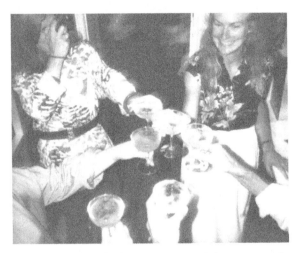

Twenty-first birthday party with co-workers

Chapter 7
Fifth Chakra - Finding Your Voice

Your fifth chakra, also known as your throat chakra, is located in your neck and throat region, and influences your thyroid gland, neck, and ears. Your fifth chakra is connected to communication, creativity, and self expression. The color associated with this chakra is blue, and its difficult aspect is lying. Speaking and listening are both aspects of your fifth chakra. When your fifth chakra is closed, you don't express your feeling or needs, and you're unable to hear expressions of the feelings and needs of others.

With a healthy and open fifth chakra, you are able to fully express yourself verbally and in writing. You speak your truth with compassion and state your boundaries with ease. You can sing or chant without embarrassment, whether you consider yourself skilled or not. You're able to release sounds that express your feelings without words. You're also a compassionate and attentive listener, and have the ability to hold space for others to speak their truth.

Sound Healing

Learning to express verbally can be challenging for those who have used silence as a survival skill. In the beginning, feelings of embarrassment or shame may accompany verbal expression in a healing context. Healing work that uses sound as a way of expressing feelings is a wonderful way to begin opening the throat chakra. A safe space can be created where any sound can be released without worry or concern about who might hear it. Opening the throat chakra often starts with coughing, choking, or gagging. Do not be alarmed by this, as it is a normal part of the process. Stay with the coughing sensations and your throat will begin to clear. Often, the first sounds that come out are unintelligible growls or soft humming. With practice and encouragement, the sounds can be expanded and can come into full expression. The release of energy that happens with sounding can be enormous and very healing. Giving voice to long-suppressed emotions has the effect of clearing space inside yourself to invite in something new. A continuing practice of sound healing will support the ongoing health and opening of your throat chakra and allow a flow of stored or blocked energy to leave your body.

Writing is also an expression of your throat chakra. Keeping your recovery journal is your first step toward clearing your throat chakra, and you began that process in the first chapter. Finding your voice is the second step in clearing and healing your throat chakra. The combination of sounding and writing will begin to create a powerful practice for your recovery journey.

Sharing Yourself with Others

If you have been very introverted, beginning to share yourself verbally with others may feel very scary and unsafe. Begin with someone you trust, and ask them to hold a safe space in which you can share something about yourself without being judged. Sharing about your recovery journey is a great way to begin to lift yourself out of shame and guilt. Alternatively, you may wish to share a story from your childhood. The important thing is to begin sharing yourself in order to practice a new skill, that of expressing yourself verbally.

Writing stories about your life and sharing them is another way to begin to express yourself as a practice. I would recommend writing true stories about something that happened to you in your past. This can be approached as writing memoirs or autobiographical stories. It can be a fun, powerful, creative exercise in self-expression.

Personal Story: *The Lion and The Cat*

I was guided to move to Auburn, CA in 2005, to live on my mom's property and work in her business as a massage therapist. It was there that I met a woman named Sally. She came for a massage, we made a nice connection, and I learned that she receives direct guidance from her Spirit Teachers. After giving her a massage for the second time, she asked if she could speak to me privately after the session. "The Spirit Teachers want me to ask you about something, but I'm not really clear what it is," she said. "Was there something going on in my second chakra?" she asked next. I usually shared the information that I felt from a person's energy system, but in this case, I did not feel anything extreme while I was working on her. There was *something*, however. "I felt some energy in your second chakra, but it wasn't anything specific," I said. She continued to ask me questions, prompted by the Spirit Teachers, and finally I asked her, "Have you been sexually abused?" Her reply was yes. It was beginning to dawn on me what this was about. I told her about the therapeutic internal healing modality I was learning about called sacred spot therapy, and she said, "YES, that is what they want me to have!" I balked a bit, saying I had not actually done this work professionally before, but that I was trained in it. She asked if I felt ready to do it, and feeling the guidance of Spirit, I said yes. We set a date that day, based on the guidance of her Spirit Teachers.

I read through all my materials in preparation for the session. Because my healing space was a room in a day spa, we needed to work on a Sunday when the spa was closed and no one else was around. I prepared the room and welcomed Sally into the sacred space. We began the session, and the things she told me as the session unfolded were not for the faint of heart.

Sally told the story of her mother, a dark shaman and mentally unbalanced woman, now in a nursing home. Sally was the youngest of several children, and she told me her mother hated her. When she was young, and the older kids were at school, her mother would abuse her in many ways and tried time and again to steal her life force. When the older siblings came home, her mother would pretend to treat her kindly, and would not have her do any chores. The older children resented her for that. Her mother was a gardener, and Sally felt she used the earth and water elements to work her dark magic.

Sally had not had a relationship in ten years, and had gotten herpes from her last partner. She had terrible outbreaks on a regular basis, and the Spirit Guides directed her to three essential oils that we were to use in the session: Rose, Melissa, and Frankincense. I mixed the essential oils liberally into the base oil we were using.
Working directly inside her yoni (vagina), I turned my finger down towards her rectum, and as I did so, the abuse story spilled out along with her rage, anger, and

terror. "My mother was gardening outside one day, and had me playing in the dirt. She shapeshifted into a tiger and raped me anally with her finger. It was as if I was being attacked by a tiger!" she cried. As I continued to press down with my finger, she released more fear and rage and horror. I encouraged her to breathe deeply. As she calmed, I told her that a spirit tiger was there in the room and that he wanted to help her. He leapt up onto the table, and lay right down on top of her, heart to heart, licking her face.

It was then that I shared with Sally what I had been through the night before. I had driven a six hour round trip in a snowstorm to put down my very sick sixteen-year-old cat, Pooky, the most beloved pet of my life. I asked her if her little inner child would like to play with Pooky in order to help heal the terror. (He looked just like an orange lion when he was still healthy.) I called upon Pooky's spirit, and he came to help. I felt so blessed to have his presence with me again. She told me he came right into her heart.

The next time I spoke to Sally, she told me that the Spirit Teachers were very happy with the progress she made, and that one session should be enough. She hasn't had a herpes outbreak since. This session was special to me in many ways. It showed me the incredible power of the work I was trained in. It also showed me that all I really need to do is create and hold the most powerful, safe, sacred space I can, and the rest will unfold perfectly. The afterlife connection with Pooky was precious to my grieving heart.

~

Learning to Listen

Perhaps you're more of an extrovert, and have no problem expressing yourself verbally. Perhaps you've spent much of your life complaining, telling others all about the drama in your life, and generally placing blame outside of yourself in a very expressive way. If this is the case, your task is to learn to listen to others. Your fifth chakra opening practice will be to hear what others have to say without thinking about how you're going to respond or defend your position. Attentive, compassionate listening is as important a skill as speaking your truth.

Exercise 5-1: Telling Your Personal Story

This exercise can be done either verbally or in writing, or both. I recommend that you choose the least comfortable method, or better yet, go with the option of both. For the writing portion, simply pour out your story on paper or on a computer, in whatever way it wants to come out. Just barf it up. Go all the way back to your childhood, as far back as you remember, and write about the things that come up in your memory. Don't be concerned about how it might sound to another for now; just allow the floodgates to open and the flow of information to pour out. This first draft of your personal story has the potential of being a very cathartic release. Whatever feelings come up as you write, take the time to feel them and be with them. You may find yourself laughing and crying as you write, and many other feelings may surface as well.

For the verbal portion of the exercise, find someone who is willing to hold a safe, non-judgmental space for you to tell your story. You can either read what you have written, or you can deliver your story from your memories. Ask the person holding space for you to simply listen without comment or gestures, allowing you to fully express all that is inside of you wanting to come out.

If you like, you can refine your written story further. From the first draft, revise the story into a more readable form, or make it more exciting and dramatic. Short stories of your life, like those that are included in this book, are also a wonderful way of sharing yourself with others.

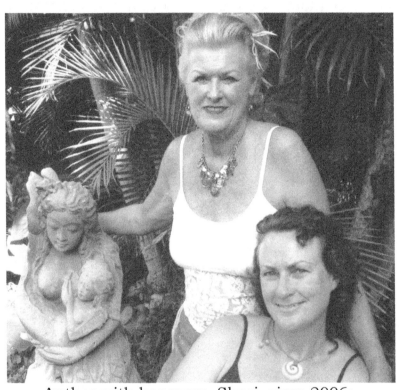

Author with her mom, Shari, circa 2006;
starting a new life on Maui.

Chapter 8
Sixth Chakra - Visualizing a New Future

Your sixth chakra, also known as your third eye, is located in the center of your forehead and influences your pineal gland. Your sixth chakra is connected to your inner vision, insight, intuition, and imagination. The color associated with this chakra is indigo, and its difficult aspect is illusion.

When your third eye is closed, you do not have access to your intuition or your insight. Your imagination is the source of subconscious symbolism and archetypal identity, and without it, you cut yourself off from a deep wellspring of rich information. If your third eye is too open, you may find it challenging to connect with others as you turn your full attention to your own inner visions.

With a healthy and open sixth chakra, you have a fully developed inner landscape that you can freely explore via your imagination. Visualization comes easily, and from this place of inner vision, you can receive insight and information that can help and guide you in your daily life. With this building block, you begin to prepare yourself for interaction with the divine aspects within you. Within this inner landscape, you can explore all aspects of yourself, your personality, your shadow sides, and the archetypal energies that are available to you for your healing and recovery. Cultivating the ability to visualize is an important component of the conscious manifestation of your reality.

The Inner Marriage

We all carry various archetypes inside of us that we're bringing forth, and you can consciously work with these archetypes to help you heal and to manifest your desires. Whether you are occupying a male or female body or have a gender-fluid or transgendered identity, you carry both an inner masculine aspect and an inner feminine aspect. These aspects can assist you in many ways, and may, at various times, represent mother and father, husband and wife, brother and sister, or any other masculine/feminine combination that you can imagine. The inner marriage is an intentional healing of these energies within you to invite balance, awareness, and integration.

Intention, Manifestation and Co-Creation

The Universal Law of Attraction, according the teachings of Abraham-Hicks Publications, states "that which is like unto itself is drawn." In other words, what you think about is what you create and become. This law is in effect whether you are aware of it or not, and whether you believe in it or not. Once you've mastered the art of using your imagination, you can use its power to consciously create that which you want to draw into your life. Often, you must overcome a lifetime of conditioning about what you think and how you speak. Like so many of the exercises in this book, it's a practice. That means that it both *takes practice,* and that it is an *exercise* (i.e., an ongoing practice). An exercise can also be defined as something one does to get in shape. The practices you are working with in this book are a way of creating new habits to replace old habits that no longer serve you; in effect, "getting in shape" mentally, emotionally, and spiritually.

That which one gives thought to *with emotion* is drawn even more powerfully. An important component is the expectation and belief that you will actually receive what you want. You can choose to wallow in self pity and whine about how unfortunate you are, thereby creating more of the same, or you can make a practice of thinking of and speaking about only about what you want in your life, as if you already have it. Rather than reiterating "what is," you can tell a new story.

Intention is a powerful part of the manifestation and co-creation process. In fact, it is the basis and foundation of all that happens in your life. At times, it may seem as though you intend one thing and experience another, which is why it's so important to dive deeply into your subconscious beliefs and unconscious behaviors. They can tend to contradict your intentions in ways that you are not fully aware of.

You may only co-create for yourself, never for another. The truth is, you can't change anyone except yourself anyway. However, the changes you make in yourself affect every other being through the web of energy that connects all of us. Once you take full responsibility for changing yourself only, it can be a real relief to let go of the need to try to effect change in others. As you make positive changes in yourself, others often react differently to you and sometimes choose to make positive changes in their own lives. You can have your greatest influence by showing up as a positive example and role model without expectations and projections on others.

There is a simple formula for co-creation and manifestation that looks like this:

Intention + Emotion + Allowing + Action = Results

We will break the formula down into further specific steps in the exercise called "The Manifestation Process."

What Do You *Really* Want?

Every one of us has the power and ability to create exactly what we want in our lives. Being able to visualize or imagine what you want is the first step to creating it. For many people, this is the hardest part; the figuring out of what it is that they want in their lives. Sometimes there are core beliefs that hold you back from believing that you can receive what you want or that you deserve to receive what you want. As you work with the practices in this book, you can slowly unwind the core beliefs that keep you thinking small. As your self-love rises, and your ability to visualize increases, you set yourself up for a life *beyond your wildest dreams!*

Exercise 6-1: Dreaming Your Desire

(bonus audio at amritagrace.com/reclaim)

This exercise requires a deep, meditative, relaxed state. Set aside some quiet time, turn off your phone, and make sure you won't be disturbed for at least half an hour. You may sit with a straight back, or lie down if you like, as long as lying down does not make you want to sleep. Some inspiring, relaxing instrumental music in the background is nice if desired. Have a pad of drawing paper and some colored pens or pencils nearby for when you come back from your dream journey.

Begin to breathe deeply, into your belly, slowly releasing each breath and taking in the next inhalation without pausing. Continue the deep belly breathing, letting the music soothe and relax you. Your breath will be an important part of the process, so keep part of your awareness on the deep, slow breathing. Now, imagine that you're traveling to a place where there are no limitations on what you can have in your life. What would a place like that look like to you? Perhaps there is a giant catalog that you can order from, with descriptions of the things you enjoy. Perhaps it's a scene from a movie or a childhood book, an imaginary place of dream fulfillment. Now that you are in this place, know that you can let your imagination run wild and free. With the freedom to choose anything you want, what will YOU choose? Continue to breathe and relax and allow whatever feelings or images that arise to just flow. Notice what shows up and how you feel about it.

In this imaginary place, where you can have your life exactly as you wish it, let your mind wander and unveil your deepest desires. If it's a partner you desire, visualize the details of his or her physical form and personality traits. See yourself interacting with your new partner and being treated like a king or queen. If it's a house, see it exactly as you want it, not limited by what you think you can afford or where you think you have to live. Stay with the visualization for as long as you like, and when you feel complete, write down or draw your desires on the paper.

Exercise 6-2: The Manifestation Process

The following steps can be used for manifesting your desires, once you have determined what they are.

- Set intention from a pure heart. Make sure you're

79

only co-creating for yourself from a place of positive energy. Use positive statements rather than stating what you don't want. If you know what you don't want, you can turn that around into a statement of what you do want. Be very specific. Write them down if you like, and post them where you can see them every day.

- Speak the intention out loud. If you like, go to a powerful place outdoors where you feel the magic of nature, or create some ceremony around your decree.

- Don't limit the universe by specifying HOW it is to be achieved, simple focus on the WHAT.

- Charge your intention with emotion. SEE and FEEL yourself receiving it and feel the joyful, grateful sensation of having it now.

- As best as you can, know and believe you will receive what you have asked for. Notice what kind of limiting beliefs come up around this.

- Don't be attached to a particular form or way that you might receive your intention. It may come in an unexpected way. Be open to infinite possibilities and the "law of grace," which will deliver what you want in the best and most expedient way possible.

- Release it fully. Let it go completely.

- Take action steps if appropriate, without pushing or forcing.

- Allow the process to unfold in its own way. Receive what is coming toward you.

- This may be the most important step of all: find gratitude for all that you already have. Then, the manifestation process simply becomes a request for "more, please"!

This process should be approached with immense respect. If you co-create and then change your mind, chances are you will still receive what you asked for. If you ask for healing (i.e., in a relationship), it may come in the form of painful and difficult process. At first this can be very disconcerting.

If you find that you have limiting beliefs emerging which have been operating under the surface, you may need to address and unwind those beliefs as part of the manifestation process.

Exercise 6-3: Meeting Your Inner Masculine (for all genders)

Create some time for yourself where you will not be disturbed for twenty to thirty minutes. Make yourself comfortable and close your eyes. Go to your personal inner sanctuary. When you feel a sense of safety and relaxation, invite your inner masculine to reveal himself. Witness whatever shows up from a neutral place, allowing him to reveal himself in whatever form he appears to you. Invite him into a dialog, asking him what he needs from you in order to feel acknowledged and integrated. Give him time to communicate in his own way. If you are a more visual person, his needs may be communicated in images and gestures rather than words. The first time I invited my inner masculine to appear, he showed up as monster covered in brown sludge. The sludge quickly melted away, and that showed me just how deeply buried he had been inside me.

This is an opportunity to experience masculine energy as safe, healing, loving, and non-sexual. Ask him if he has any needs or requests. Tell him what you need from him. The masculine holds space, witnesses without judgment, and creates safety. Whether you're a man or a woman, you need your inner masculine aspects for balance. When you feel complete, thank him and let him know you appreciate him.

Exercise 6-4: Meeting Your Inner Feminine (for all genders)

This exercise will be just like meeting your inner masculine, only this time you will meet your inner feminine. From your personal inner sanctuary, invite your inner feminine to reveal herself and her needs and requests. Communicate to her your needs from her, and be sure to release her with appreciation and gratitude when you feel complete. As an additional exercise, you may wish to bring your inner masculine and feminine together and invite them to interact and integrate.

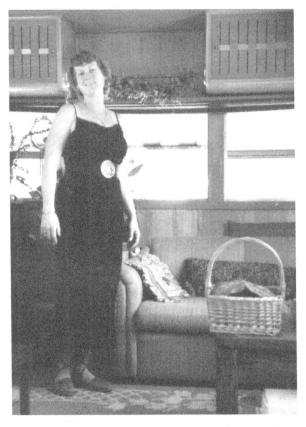

Just over a year into recovery, solid on the path.

Chapter 9
Seventh Chakra - Connecting to Your Divine Self

Your seventh chakra, also known as your crown, is located on the top of your head and influences your pituitary gland and your cerebral cortex. Your seventh chakra is connected to pure awareness, divine unity, and spiritual union. The color associated with this chakra is purple, and its difficult aspects are attachment and ignorance. When your crown is closed, you do not have access to your spiritual guidance. You have closed yourself off from "heavenly" input. You may feel you're all alone in the world and that you're not connected to anyone or anything.

When you are healthy and open in your crown, you open yourself to guidance from your higher selves, ascended masters, teachers, spirit guides, animal totems, and your higher power, whatever that means for you. These protecting forces are always around you, ready to assist if you ask. However, they will not assist you against your free will. With an open crown, you have the ability to channel divine wisdom, healing, and love through your being. You may speak this divine wisdom or perhaps lay your hands upon yourself or another with healing intention. You begin to see yourself as a divine being in your own right, acknowledging that you're simply having a brief human experience so that your soul can learn and grow. You can begin to grasp the edges of the concept of "eternity," giving a much larger context to this human life you are currently experiencing. You begin to see the divine being in others. You feel less and less of a need to project your stories and fantasies on others, allowing everyone to just be who they are.

Personal Story: *Black Angels in Gray Hoodies*

March 27, 2009 was a day filled with sadness and racial tension in the San Francisco Bay Area. In the days preceding, four police officers had been shot and killed by a paroled criminal, two of whom were pulling him over for a traffic violation. As is common in one of the most liberal areas in the US, a civil rights rally had been held the day before for the criminal, proclaiming with signs that the man had become a criminal *because* of racism.

On Friday, March 27th, thousands of police officers turned out for a memorial funeral march across the Bay Bridge. My sister Cyndi was witness to this as she crossed the Bay Bridge in the opposite direction on her way to work. At her workplace, the mood was somber and depressed. Many declared their shame and embarrassment to live in a community where such a thing could happen.

I was staying at Cyndi's house, having traveled from Maui for a weekend workshop in San Francisco. I decided to take the BART rapid transit train into the City from her home south of San Francisco. Before coming to the mainland from Maui, I had studied the BART website so that I could navigate with some semblance of competence, and I left myself plenty of time to buffer any miscalculations or moments of disorientation. Once on BART and satisfied I was heading in the right direction, I decided to listen to my voicemail. I kept trying, but eventually gave up because the background noise on the train was too loud.

I got off at my stop in the heart of the SOMA district in the City, and walked with ease to my destination. From there, I dove right in to the workshop and did not think about anything else. At the end of the evening, having asked someone to walk me to the BART station, I hopped on the train and went into my pack for my cell phone. I didn't find it, so I dug through it a couple more times, then thought back to the last time I saw it. The last thing I remembered was being mildly frustrated about not being able to hear my voicemail and giving up. I also had a vague thought that I had never heard my phone ring during the workshop, and I was pretty sure I had not turned it off.

I decided I would check in the backpack that I had left in the workshop space the next morning. I took a slight track through the idea that I may have left it on the train earlier, but it seemed unlikely. If I had, there was little I would be able to do about it tonight. I was facing a short night of sleep and a fourteen hour workshop day on Saturday. I weighed in my mind how much priority I needed to give it, and decided it was not worth worrying about. I drove to my sister's house from the BART station, and when I got home, she was waiting up for me.

Cyndi told me she had left a little present for me on my pillow. I was baffled, and she went into the room to get it. She came out with my phone. I took a slight step backwards. "Whoa, how on earth.......?" I exclaimed. "Did I leave it on the BART train?" She was nodding, and had a transcendent look on her face. I knew she had a story to tell, and the story that unfolded was nothing short of a miracle. Here's what she told me:

"It was late in the day at my office, and I got a call from your cell number. I answered it, and a man was speaking. There was a strange noise in the background, and I abruptly hung up, a little startled. I decided to call back, wondering what the heck was going on. I called back and the man who answered said he had found the phone on the BART train. I was starting to freak out. Who was this strange man, and how did he get my sister's phone? Where was my sister?

"I asked him where he found the phone and where he was heading. He said he found it on the BART and was on his way to Oakland. I asked if I could meet him somewhere and pick up the phone, as I knew you would be missing it. He said he was heading to the MacArthur BART station, which is in the most racially charged part of Oakland. My levels of adrenaline were climbing, but I knew I needed to get that phone. If it was my phone, I would be spinning out and in a panic. I figured that must be how you were feeling.

"I asked the man his name, and he said it was Charlie. I asked him how I would know him, and he said he was a black man wearing a gray hoodie. I took a deep breath and wondered if this was a setup. He said he was going to pick up his daughter from school and I relaxed by a small degree. He must be okay if he is a dad, I thought.

"By now, Charlie felt like my new best friend. I made arrangements to leave work early, even though I had gotten a lecture that morning from my boss about not leaving early. This was an emergency. My co-workers were assisting me with directions to the MacArthur BART, and advising me to just leave and not worry about the boss. I could not wait to get out of that place, where the somber mood and funereal sadness had just about drained me dry.

"I called my husband to let him know what I was doing,

but did not dare disclose where I was going or who I was meeting. With his protective nature and lifelong experience of living in the Bay Area, he would have forbidden it. I had to keep it from him. He helped me figure out how to operate the GPS unit, and I was on my way with more than a little trepidation.

"As I pulled up to the curb, I called Charlie on your phone again to let him know what I was driving. He answered, and again I wondered how on earth I would find him with a description that fit about 80% of the population of the MacArthur BART station. As I told him what I was driving and what I looked like, he said "Oh, I see you, that's me with the pink stroller." The next level of my wall of fear and trepidation crumbled.

"He came to the window and handed me the phone. I thanked him profusely and asked him if he would accept a little something for his trouble. He thought about it and then refused. I told him his little girl was just beautiful and that what he had done was a great deed. He went on his way and I thought to call him once more to thank him, and at that moment, I realized that I had no way to reach him anymore. I turned toward home.

"I tried to figure out how to get a hold of you, Amrita. I was sure you would be worried sick about your phone, I know I would have! I thought about trying to find your car at the BART station and leaving a note on it, or finding the number to reach you in the workshop, but I did not know where to begin to find a way to reach you.

"I could not sleep. I could not stand the suspense of waiting until morning to tell you how your phone came to be at the house. I thought, maybe she'll just think she left it here, and it won't be any big deal. I have to tell her tonight, no matter how late she gets in. The one thing that I can't figure out is how he chose me to call. I was not the last person you called or who called you; in fact, I was way down on the recent calls list!"

That night, Cyndi told me the story three times in rapid succession. I just smiled when she told me she was sure I would be freaking out. I told her that I live my life in trust these days, and that I am always taken care of. This was a prime example.

Over the next twenty-four hours, as I let the story integrate into my being, I realized that it was not at all about me or my phone. It was a miracle involving a black angel in a gray hoodie, come to deliver a message or two to my sister Cyndi. I was simply a cog in the delivery vehicle for the Universe's angel messages.

Cyndi's faith in humanity has been restored. She has witnessed a process of letting go of the illusion of control and of the concept of pronoia, *the suspicion that the Universe is a conspiracy on your behalf.* I've been subscribing to the concept of pronoia for some time now, and I love seeing it demonstrated so dramatically. Cyndi also pointed out that with Obama as president, there is new hope for the dissolving of racial tension. I hope she's right. I think it starts inside of each of us; as we heal ourselves, we heal the collective.

Thank you Charlie, my black angel in a gray hoodie!

~

Embodying the Divine

"Transpersonal" is a word used to describe a state that is beyond the personality of this human life, and delves into the perception of yourself and others as divinity incarnate. You can share transpersonal space with another by having an agreement to do so, aided by creating sacred space and using your intention. Perhaps you have a particular archetype that you feel called to work with, such as Aphrodite, the goddess of love; or Kwan Yin, the goddess of compassion. Using your intention, you can call forth the qualities of these archetypes (and many others) to come into your energy field and inform you directly of the qualities they bring. Divine embodiment is generally best done in a ceremonial setting, creating sacred space and time.

Compassion and Unconditional Love
for Self and Others

You cannot truly love another until you have learned to love yourself. The same is true of compassion. After nearly a decade of recovery from sexual addiction, I experienced the key to the whole process as being self-love. Every step on the path was leading me to loving myself. Loving myself created self–compassion automatically as part of the process. It's been a long journey from fear, control, contraction, and unconsciousness to this place of self love, and yet I see now that it has been the only journey I could take if I wished to be free of my wounding.

Being able to look in the mirror and like what I see... knowing that I have so much to offer and having that reflected to me by others day after day... being able to receive and accept the gifts that others offer... enjoying my own company even when I feel lonely... being gentle with myself when I make mistakes, these are some of the gifts that come with self-love. The most precious gift of all was having my beloved appear in my life after years of being single and so strongly desiring a life partner who could match the person I had become. Ultimately, we attract that which we are, and my commitment to healing and self-love drew to me a man who met and exceeded everything I wanted and had asked for in a partner.

Individual Spiritual Path

All paths lead to the ONE. If I were to state my concept of "religion," that's what I would say. Religions are the creation of man, and seem to have less and less validity as the world accelerates in its transformational process. Each one of us creates our own individual spiritual path, even if we're a member of a particular religion. It's human nature to take what we like from what we learn, and release what we don't like. Even very strict dogmas have only limited influence on the free will of the human mind. We each form our own moral code, and from that place of inner integrity, we adapt our spiritual path to fit what works for us, and continue to refine and create that path throughout our lives. At times, we may go through sweeping changes in our spiritual paths. At other times, we may feel very steady.

If you feel that you have had a particular religion imposed upon you, especially when you were a child, I invite you to release whatever does not serve you about that religion, along with any guilt or shame, and begin to create exactly what you want in your spiritual path. It is perfectly natural and normal to take what you like from several different doctrines and meld it into something that works best for you as an individual. If you feel drawn to a particular path, take the time to explore what it offers and embrace only those parts of it that you like. Creating your own spiritual path is like creating a beautiful painting on a blank canvas. Following a particular religion because someone told you that you had to is more like a paint-by-numbers picture. You have free will and personal choice, and are an empowered being, fully capable of defining exactly what is best for YOU in every moment.

Creating Sacred Space

Creating sacred space is a way of informing your subconscious that a special time and mood is required. The easiest way to create sacred space is to use your intention. You can simply state that you are entering sacred space and it will be so. Or, you can get more elaborate by setting up an altar with sacred objects, calling in your guides and angels, and using sage or incense to purify the space.

From sacred space, you can move more easily into non-ordinary states of consciousness, such as a meditative state. Your rational mind can relax, which gives you access to your right brain functions of imagery and intuition. Sacred space can be created anywhere, indoors or out. The most important thing to remember is that your time in sacred space should not be interrupted by phones, children, pets, or other distractions.

Exercise 7-1: The World-Wide Hug

Create your sacred space in whatever way you like. Imagine that you are no longer bound by the confines of your body. You are growing larger and larger, and the earth is getting smaller and smaller, until you can hold it in your arms like a beach ball. Take the earth into your arms and imagine that you are a mother to all the creatures who live on her. Imagine you can send them all the love and compassion in your heart, and that this will make their lives immeasurably better. Take some time to send them your love and compassion, remembering to include yourself in the showering of love. Continue until you feel yourself overflowing with gratitude for this opportunity to express your love to all creatures.

Exercise 7-2: Meeting Your Guides

Create your sacred space in whatever way you like. Each of us has a number of guardian angels, spirit guides, and animal helpers that support our human process from other realms. If you would like to meet some or all of yours, you need only make your intention known and then receive their help and guidance. You may ask for specific information about them (such as what your animal totem is) or you may simply trust that they have been chosen for you by a loving higher power who wants you to receive your highest options.

A meditative state is the best way to make contact with your guides, as they will often give you symbolic guidance in the form of feelings, inner images, or a sense of knowing. You can go to your inner sanctuary if you like, and ask for your guides to introduce themselves to you.

Each of us has a different way of perceiving our guides, so just allow whatever presents itself to be just right. It may be an image that comes to you, or a feeling of safety. Many people receive direct, clear guidance from their guides, while others experience a more subtle form of contact. If you're clear in your intention that you want to receive support from your guides, trust that the support will come in whatever form is going to serve you best.

Exercise 7-3: Embracing Your Divinity

Create your sacred space in whatever way you like. This exercise can be done alone, while looking in a mirror, or with another person. When working with another, sit or stand facing the other person, and gently gaze into each other's left (receptive) eye. Allowing your gaze to soften and looking past their personality, see the other, or yourself, as they truly are: a divine being, a god or goddess. As you notice and cultivate this quality of divinity within yourself, you begin to notice it more readily in others around you. A lovely acknowledgment of the divine in another is the use of the word and gesture "Namasté." With your hands folded in prayer position and your thumbs pressed into your heart chakra, bow to the person before you while saying Namasté. It means "the divine in me recognizes and honors the divine in you."

Use the same process with yourself in a mirror, including the Namasté.

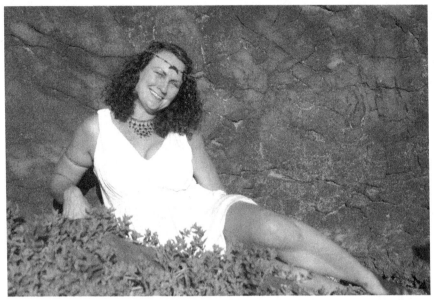

Just prior to the first (2009) edition of this book. Fully recovered and ready to assist others on their healing paths. Aphrodite embodied!

Photo by David Bolles

Chapter 10
Further Healing and Integration

Somatic Sexual Healing

There is a whole new generation of healers who address the second chakra (sexual center) in a therapeutic context, assisting people in releasing stored energies that are no longer serving their highest options. It's not necessary to have a history of abuse or trauma to receive benefit from this type of healing. We are all impacted to some degree by the collective sexual shadow that is perpetuated in our society through pornography, religious dogma, and the use of sex to advertise all manner of goods and services. It's not just the commercialization – it's the repression wrought by the idea that sex is not a wholesome, beautiful, natural part of life. Imagine sexual *innocence* in advertising. If we actually were a sexually healthy society, sex would no longer hold a manipulative role – we would just enjoy it for the pure, creative, life force energy that it is.

For those with a history of sexual abuse, this kind of healing work can produce miracles. Shame, guilt, rage, and anger are given a safe outlet as the healer creates and holds sacred, neutral space in which you can deeply breathe and give voice and sounds to the long-stored emotions.

Those who offer this kind of healing work are trained to create safe, sacred energetic containers in which people of all genders can get in touch with any energies or emotions that might be stored in their second chakras, or anywhere in their energy fields and bodies. In the safe, neutral space, they can release abuse and trauma, rage, shame, and guilt with breath, movement, and sounds. The internal spaciousness and freedom that can be created from this kind of release can be consciously filled with whatever you choose for yourself. You may also find that a great deal of energy has been freed up that you can use in new ways in your life.

If you choose to seek out this kind of work, it's important to find someone to work with that you feel really safe with in order to confront these hidden and taboo memories and buried emotions. There is a wide range of styles of practitioners in this unregulated field, and some are more educated, trained, and experienced than others.

Your Body is a Sacred Temple

As you release shame and guilt and learn to honor your body as a sacred temple, you reclaim your birthright as an ecstatic spiritual sexual being. Integrating your sexuality into your whole being will feel brand new to most people who have previously compartmentalized this aspect of their lives. Love and acceptance of your body, just the way it is, soon follows. A strong desire to lovingly care for your body is a natural result of reclaiming your sexual wholeness. Healthy food, regular exercise, good sleep, a balance of work and play, and addressing other compulsions in your life may also result from a steady, ongoing healing path.

Sexual Sobriety & Abstinence

It's one thing for alcoholics to know when they are sober. It's quite another for someone recovering from sexual wounding or addiction to know when they are practicing sobriety. Sexual sobriety and abstinence are not the same thing. Abstinence is a total refrain from sexual activity. Sobriety is a refrain from sexual acting-out behavior. The knowledge and understanding of sexual sobriety comes with time and healing and with an increase in personal integrity. It also comes with ability to "track" yourself and be completely honest with yourself. When you are willing to witness your behaviors and identify them honestly, you can make healthy decisions about your actions before you take them.

A period of abstinence may be a healthy choice for anyone who is healing from sexual wounding. When you take time for yourself, without the influence of anyone else's energy, you have an opportunity for deeper healing and a more accelerated path to self love and self acceptance. You also give yourself the opportunity to create intimacy with yourself and sexual sovereignty, both valuable qualities to take into your next relationship. A period of abstinence can bring great clarity.

Reclaiming Your Sexual Wholeness

How does a sexually whole being show up in the world? Let's examine the word *integrity*. *Integrity* may be seen as "the quality of having a sense of honesty and truthfulness in regard to the motivations for one's actions." Integrity with your sexual energy is the first indicator of a sexually whole being. I consider myself to be a fully recovered and sexually whole being, so I will use myself as an example.

My interpretation of integrity with sexual energy is that I am aware of my sexual energy and how I'm using it at all times. I am using my tools to manage it so that I don't use it to manipulate or control others. If I do slip in my integrity, which I occasionally do, being human, I notice it as soon as possible and make appropriate amends where needed.

I monitor myself and my behavior in all potentially sexual situations for any vestiges of compulsive behavior. If I do see something that echoes my previous addictive behavior, I notice it with compassion and I never beat myself up. I instantly forgive myself, feel any feelings that come up around it, correct any mistakes, and learn from the experience.

I care about my sexual health and have regular gynecological checkups. Prior to engaging in a monogamous relationship, I had regular testing for STD's, practiced safe sex at all times, and had conversations with my potential partners about their sexual histories and mine. I disclosed any dis-eases or concerns I may have had before engaging sexually. As I gained sexual sobriety, I came to have very high standards in my intimate partners, and expected them to be as concerned about their sexual health as I am about mine.

I do not take on other people's moral or religious ideologies if they do not fit with my belief system. I look inside myself for what is appropriate for me, right now. I see how relationship forms are changing and evolving from the traditional monogamous relationship, and I honor all forms of relationship, even if I don't choose them for myself.

I love and accept my body, every part of it. When I look in

the mirror, I like what I see, and sometimes, it even takes my breath away! People often tell me that I am beautiful and this feels wonderful to me. I understand that what they are seeing is my inner beauty, my love and acceptance of myself, and the powerful light that shines from my being. It feels great and it's more powerful than any kind of cosmetics or hairstyle.

I have been comfortable with being single, which meant being celibate at times. During times of celibacy, I kept my second chakra energy moving and open, so that I had access to my creativity and life force energy. I don't ever want to shut down my sexual energy and cut myself off from my Shakti (the feminine life force energy).

I have a regular practice of self-pleasuring and sexual loving with myself. I do not use vibrators which can desensitize the delicate vaginal tissues; instead I use specially designed wands made of lucite, crystal or blown glass. I enter myself with reverence and respect.

Ultimately, reclaiming my sexual wholeness paved the way for a truly healthy, deeply fulfilling relationship with my beloved life partner, a man who is also whole and healed and able to meet me as an equal as well as support me in the full expression of who I am and who I am becoming.

Personal Story: *Manifesting My Beloved*

I had taken every step in the manifestation process, made my lists of qualities, and done my healing work over the course of several years, and I was *still* single. I hopefully posted profiles to several dating sites, and kept my mind and heart open. Eventually, I let it all go, removed my profiles and closed the dating site accounts, and just focused on my relationship with myself. I still stayed alert to any possibilities that might appear, and investigated any leads.

I felt a strong urging to attend a weekend sacred sexuality conference in Sedona in 2008, and I followed that intuition. It was there that I met Apollo. He had been serving as an apprentice at the Sedona Temple, the organization that was hosting the conference, for the past month. I felt very drawn to him, and also a little intimidated.

A woman friend of mine who was also attending the conference revealed to me that she had interacted with Apollo, and she found him quite approachable. She told me that he was polyamorous, and that he had a wife and several girlfriends that he dated in his hometown of Minneapolis. I was attracted and intrigued.

I received another strong intuition to stay after the conference for a four-day workshop in the Temple. I decided to see if I could easily make those arrangements, and if so, I would take that as a green light to stay. I effortlessly changed my plane ticket, made arrangements for someone to take my rental car to the airport in my place, and stayed for the workshop.

I learned that Apollo would also be attending the workshop, and introduced myself to him. I knew that there were more women than men participating, and I really wanted to have an opportunity to work with a man in some of the processes. (At least, that was what I told myself.) When I learned there would be a partnered Shamanic Breathwork exercise, I asked Apollo to partner with me and he agreed.

As part of the exercise, Apollo and I made agreements about how to participate. I was to be the first to do the breathwork, and he would watch over me and provide support as needed. Just before I pulled the blindfold mask over my eyes, he said, "Oh and by the way, I'm very attracted to you!" With that, I went into my inner journey.

As the workshop progressed, we found time to talk and cuddle. He told me about his polyamorous lifestyle, and how well it worked for him. He and his wife lived with her other "husband," who was like a brother to him. They each had additional lovers, all of which were disclosed to the others, and had been living happily in this arrangement for several years.

I decided that this man was worth risking my heart for. Even though I did not identify as polyamorous, I was willing to explore the possibilities of being one of his girlfriends. We parted ways at the Phoenix airport utterly dazzled by the strength of our connection.

I went home to Maui and he went home to Minneapolis. We lived 4,000 miles apart, but we never let that get in the way. Apollo, being a computer programmer, had lots of skills and tools to keep us connected across the miles. We had web cameras at our home office workstations, and would see still photos of each other that were updated every few seconds as we went about our workdays. We would have hours-long video chats, and sometimes we would just leave the video chats going while we went about our days. Once, he even set it up so that I could be part of a party at his home in Minneapolis by virtue of the webcams.

We were physically separated for seven months that first time. In December of that year, he came to Hawaii to participate in a workshop that I was staffing and then to stay with me for ten days after the workshop. We became lovers after the workshop and began to build a relationship in person.

Apollo had everything I had asked for, and so much more. There was just this one thing. I had asked for a monogamous relationship. Under no circumstances would I ask him to be any different than he was, however. I decided to just stay open and keep investigating what was being presented to me.

I visited his home in Minneapolis and met his other partners. I appreciated how successfully they were engaged in their lifestyle. They invited me to come and live with them, but I was very clear that I would not be comfortable with that arrangement. We continued our long-distance relationship and stayed very close. Because of my own travels, we were able to see a great deal of each other, and our relationship deepened.

On some level I knew this man was my beloved, but I was not willing to speak, or even think it just yet. I chose to continue to hold to my clear desire to have a monogamous beloved relationship, and I did speak that. As much as I loved Apollo, I did my best to remain unattached to having him be the partner I was calling in. Apollo was very supportive and wanted me to have what was right for me, even if that could not be him. He later told me, "I didn't think it was going to be me, even though I loved you deeply. So I wanted him to come into your life. I was looking forward to meeting him - I thought he'd be a pretty amazing guy." I took the risk, kept my heart open, and allowed myself to fall deeply in love.

On a visit to Maui in 2009, and during an evening of deep connection with each other, Apollo declared me his beloved. I could hardly believe my ears. I could finally allow my full truth to come to the surface and be spoken. But how would it work? Neither of us knew, but we trusted.

Apollo returned home after that visit, and over the course of the next several weeks, he came to realize that his life in Minneapolis was coming to completion. His wonderful fourteen-year marriage was coming to the end of its cycle. He was moving to Maui.

He completed his marriage with grace and generosity, making sure that his former wife was well cared for. She legally married her other husband as soon as the divorce was final, and they continue to prosper in their relationship.

I welcomed him into my little island home, made space for him, and we began to create our new life together. I completely trusted that we would work through whatever we needed to around the monogamy vs. non-monogamy issues.

Two short years after that first breathwork session, in the very same room and during a similar breathwork process, Apollo proposed. I, of course, accepted, and we got married on Maui in December 2010, followed by a ceremony before our families on Maui in March 2011.

Apollo and I are in a monogamous relationship. Apollo chose this with me, and I am deeply grateful. When his desire to be polyamorous again came to the surface in 2015, we used our powerful communication tools and the depth of our love and connection to work through it to its conclusion. It took us nine months and a very intense underworld journey, but we came out the other side a stronger and more mature couple.

Never, ever give up. Although life is full of compromises, I urge you to explore your deepest core values and to hold true to them, no matter what the risk or potential losses, while also allowing others to find their own way and their own truth. Things are not always what they appear to be on the surface; and this story is my living, breathing proof.

~

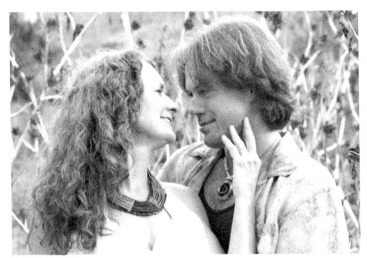

Amrita & Apollo Grace, January 2012

Our Divine Creation

We are all high spiritual energy beings who have chosen to be embodied on Earth in order to participate in the accelerated changes of the current transformational times. We are aspects of Source, of Creator. There is nowhere to look for "God" except inside ourselves, for we are the divine creators as well as the *creations* of our reality. Each of us is in the perfect place in our process. As you learn to accept yourself in this divine perfection and take full responsibility for your reality, peace and trust replace resistance and the illusion of control. Gratitude and joy replace fear and resentment. Love rules your body, mind, and heart.

I wish you abundant love, compassion, and blessings on your path of growth and healing. I acknowledge you for your courage and your willingness to receive this information. Thank you for being born, and for choosing to be alive right now.

Aloha nui loa

Amrita Grace, Maui, Hawaii
December 24, 2009

Revised August 16, 2012
Maui, Hawaii

Revised December 21, 2017
Whittier, North Carolina

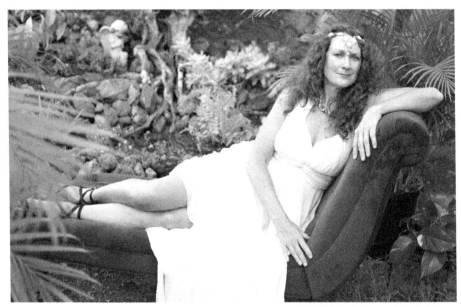

I wish you bright blessings on your path to wholeness!

Acknowledgments

From the bottom of my heart, I extend my gratitude to every person who has touched my life along its spiral path. Those who were present in my life prior to my recovery experienced a great deal of intensity and drama with me, and I appreciate how you stood by me. I want to especially thank my parents, for providing the gateway into this life, and my sisters, who helped me temper myself into a functional adult.

I give thanks to both of my former husbands, who bore the brunt of my sexual addiction, and reflected me back to myself with so much clarity. I am grateful to my abuser, for without him, I would not be the amazingly healed being that I am today.

I specifically thank my mentors and teachers, most notably Johanna Atman, Jim Hellam, Caroline Muir, Joan Heartfield, Saida Désilets, Betty Martin, Rachael Jayne Groover, Baba Dez Nichols, and David Cates. There are many others, too numerous to mention. I hope you know who you are.

I am deeply appreciative to Lisa Donnelly and Apollo Grace for their editing and proofreading efforts on the first draft of the manuscript.

I am grateful beyond words to my beloved life partner and muse, Apollo Grace, the first man in my life I have had a truly healthy intimate relationship with. And to my cherished sisters on the path: Kristine Louise, Lisa Donnelly, and Asha Stokes, I thank you for your lifetimes of support and love.

Most of all, I am deeply grateful to myself, for having the courage to forge a path of healing that was neither traditional nor mainstream.

Mahalo Nui Loa

Bibliography

There are dozens of books that have influenced my healing journey and this book. These are some of the most influential.

Auel, Jean M.
Valley of the Horses
Bantam, 2002

Bonheim, Jalaja
Aphrodite's Daughters
Fireside, 1997

Carroll, Lee
All of the Kryon channeled works
Kryon Writings

Désilets, Ph.D., Saida
Emergence of the Sensual Woman
Jade Goddess Publishing, 2006

Groover, Rachael Jayne
Powerful and Feminine
Deep Pacific Press, 2011

Hicks, Esther & Jerry
All of the Abraham channeled works
Abraham Hicks Publications

Humanity Healing Network
The Wounded Healer, 2009
www.humanityhealing.org

Judith, Anodea
Chakra Balancing Kit: A Guide to Healing and Awakening Your Energy Body
Sounds True, 2006

Kasl, Ph.D., Charlotte Davis
Women, Sex, and Addiction
Harper and Row, 1989

Muir, Caroline and Muir, Charles
Tantra: The Art of Conscious Loving
Book Baby, 1989

O'Malley, Mary
The Gift of Our Compulsions
New World Library, 2004

Stubbs, Kenneth Ray
Women of the Light: The New Sacred Prostitute
Access Publishers Network, 1994

Stubbs, Kenneth Ray & Sarah Sher
*Magdalene Unveiled: The Ancient and Modern
Sacred Prostitute (DVD)*
Secret Garden Publishing, 2006

Trimpey, Jack
*Rational Recovery: The New Cure for
Substance Addiction*
Pocket Books, 1996

Be sure to visit AmritaGrace.com/reclaim for additional complimentary resources to support your journey to wholeness.

Made in the USA
Coppell, TX
04 June 2021